PMS

THE ESSENTIAL GUIDE TO TREATMENT OPTIONS

Dr Katharina Dalton
with David Holton

Thorsons
An Imprint of HarperCollins*Publishers*

Thorsons
An Imprint of HarperCollins*Publishers*
77–85 Fulham Palace Road,
Hammersmith, London W6 8JB
1160 Battery Street,
San Francisco, California 94111-1213

Published by Thorsons 1994
10 9 8 7 6 5 4 3 2 1

A catalogue record for this book
is available from the British Library

ISBN 0 7225 3006 4

Typeset by Harper Phototypesetters Limited
Northampton, England
Printed in Great Britain by
Mackays of Chatham, Kent

CONTENTS

List of Illustrations   vi
Preface   ix
Introduction: Does PMS Exist?   xiii

PART I: WHAT IS PMS AND WHAT CAUSES IT?

1. Freedom of Choice   3
2. If It's Not PMS   18
3. What Does It Feel Like?   35
4. What Causes PMS?   42

PART II: TREATMENT METHODS

5. Self-help   59
6. Diet and PMS   69
7. Treatment Without Drugs   81
8. Over-the-Counter Medicines: Are They Any Use?   90
9. Drugs to Relieve Symptoms   104
10. Progesterone Treatment   116
11. Other Hormonal Approaches   134
12. Surgical Options   141
13. Progesterone and Conception, Pregnancy and
      Contraception   147
14. The Success Rates of Different PMS Treatments   161
15. The 'Best Buys'   175
    Glossary   181
    Further Reading   187
    Useful Addresses   188
    Index   191

LIST OF ILLUSTRATIONS

Figure
1. Severity of symptoms
2. Simple menstrual chart
3. Three menstrual charts showing different menstrual cycles and timing of symptoms
4. Japanese menstrual charts showing PMS
5. Sterilization increases PMS whether the tubes are tied, cut, clipped or cauterized
6. Controlling centres of the brain
7. Charts showing menstrual distress
8. Varying severity of PMS exacerbation in menstrual distress
9. Site and time of pain in spasmodic and congestive dysmenorrhoea
10. Charts of sufferers of spasmodic and congestive dysmenorrhoea
11. Blood progesterone levels in a normal menstrual cycle, during pregnancy and after giving birth (puerperium)
12. Sites of menopausal symptoms
13. Menstrual charts of women at the menopause
14. Proportion of physical and psychological PMS symptoms
15. PMS sufferers go from specialist to specialist
16. Dr Quack's instant PMS cures
17. Levels of oestrogen and progesterone throughout the menstrual cycle
18. Hormonal pathway from the brain to the womb
19. SHBG binding capacity in 50 patients with severe PMS and 50 controls
20. Rise in SHBG levels in PMS patients given progesterone therapy

21. Cell with progesterone receptors
22. Animals requiring progesterone receptors
23. Sites of progesterone receptors
24. Progesterone levels after large meals
25. PMS sufferers who eat breakfast
26. Overnight food gaps in women with PMS
27. Effect of three-hourly starch diet on PMS and menstrual distress
28. Symptoms of vitamin B_6 overdose
29. Depression is a disease of loss
30. Antidepressants for types of depression
31. Elephant's toes
32. Production of progesterone
33. Effect of administration of progesterone and progestogens on blood progesterone level
34. Time of starting progesterone with different lengths of menstrual cycles
35. 'Happy tampons'
36. Site for progesterone injections
37. Formulae of progesterone, a progestogen and testosterone: which compound does norethisterone resemble?
38. Menstrual chart one year after a hysterectomy
39. Incidence of PMS after a normal pregnancy and one complicated by pre-eclampsia
40. Above-average grades of 79 children 9–10 years old
41. University places gained by 'progesterone children' and controls
42. Stages of postnatal depression as it gradually changes to PMS
43. Treatments before attendance at the PMS clinic (1983 and 1993)
44. Benefit of over-the-counter medication for PMS
45. Benefit of hormone therapy plus the three-hourly starch diet for PMS
46. Benefit of alternative medicine for PMS
47. Is it PMS?
48. It's not PMS
49. It is PMS

PREFACE

This book has been written to fulfil a definite need for women searching for relief from their once-a-month miseries and sufferings. The size of this need can be gauged from the public reaction to my five-minute TV appearance one Thursday morning in January 1991. When the BBC asked for an address from which viewers could obtain further information, Wendy Holton hurriedly organized a PO Box number on the Monday. By the morning after the TV show there were already nearly 500 letters pleading for help, and within the week some 4,000 letters had arrived. This led to the foundation of PMS Help, an organization whose activities are mentioned in the last chapter. Daily, the post continues to pour in from confused, depressed and weeping women, their husbands, families and friends, both from Britain and all around the world. Nowhere, it seems, have most women yet found an answer to PMS.

I suffered from migraine since puberty, with excruciating pain in one side of my head – how I longed to just cut my head in half and be left with only the side with no pain. This migraine continued and became worse after each of my first three pregnancies, and it was only then that I realized my migraines came before periods, were absent during my pregnancies and were particularly severe within a few days of childbirth. In 1948 I was a final-year medical student and sought help from physicians, neurologists, gynaecologists and ear, nose and throat surgeons, but it was only when I met the endocrinologist Dr Raymond Greene that he appreciated the relationship of migraine to menstruation. He suggested progesterone treatment, and there followed 14 migraine-free years. This was the beginning of our work together, and it was in our publication in the *British Medical*

Journal in 1953 that the term 'Premenstrual Syndrome' was first used. Speaking on the subject at the Royal Society of Medicine in 1954, I said:

> The cost of progesterone therapy is high, but when this charge is weighed against the price in terms of human misery, suffering and injustice, it is seen as a justifiable expense opening up a new vista in Medicine.

It is indeed sad to see the human suffering and misery from PMS still continuing today. This is the first book written by an active medical practitioner who has had the unique experience of treating and observing women with PMS for over 40 years. After more than 20 years in general practice, observing the effect of menstruation on all diseases, and the effect of PMS on both the sufferer and her family, I became a consultant dealing solely with PMS and postnatal depression. Over the years I have closely followed up several hundred PMS sufferers for 10 or more years. This meant long-term study of PMS through puberty tantrums and truancy, relationship problems, contraception, pregnancies (both wanted and unwanted), and on until after the menopause and prevention of osteoporosis.

In 1985 it was decided to form an international medical society devoted to furthering research into and understanding of PMS. The Dalton Society has since held international conferences in Los Angeles, Chicago, Tulsa, Oklahoma City, San Francisco and London; the next meeting is planned for Perth, Australia, in 1994. So, work on finding the answer to PMS is continuing world-wide.

In my many travels abroad it is interesting that the questions asked at PMS meetings and TV appearances are all the same. PMS is a world-wide problem, women everywhere are searching for an answer, and the need for help is never-ending. Too many women are afraid to approach their family doctor fearing that their problem will be considered too trivial, time-wasting or 'all in the mind'.

There are over 100 options considered in this book, to treat the 150 different symptoms of PMS. I have either tried the options myself or have heard at first-hand the results of the various options which my patients have tried. All women are different, their symptoms are different in type and severity, so are their ages, lifestyles, homes, families and genetic make-up. It is not surprising that there are so many different suggestions to help individuals with what has been described as 'the world's commonest disease'. Each sufferer is individual and unique; I am sure there is an answer for each one, although inevitably the answer will be different.

The entrepreneurs, on the other hand, are aware of the gap in medicine and have rushed to offer consumers pills and potions which have never been tested. Alternative and complementary medical practitioners have also tried to fill the gap. Meanwhile, the brilliant new findings of the molecular biologists in regard to progesterone and PMS are disregarded by the medical establishment while the gynaecologists busy themselves with *in vitro* fertilization and keyhole surgery, and the psychiatrists treat these PMS problems as if they were of psychological origin, expecting them to respond to one of the ever-increasing number of new drugs for depression and anxiety.

It is my hope that this book will help women to choose the best treatment for their own particular problem. I accept that there will be some who will read this book straight through and that there will be others who will pick out the particular chapter that seems most appropriate at the moment. To help these 'dipper' readers there are many cross-references and some duplication of information.

My sincere appreciation of David Holton's valuable work in 'ghosting' this book is shown in having his name as the joint author. He has taken over from my late husband, Revd Tom Dalton, the task of converting my thoughts on PMS into an easily readable work. Those who are already familiar with my many other books will notice the difference and the younger approach he has brought. He has thrown away hundreds of commas, as well as writing several sections of the book from scratch. Thank you, David, also for your help when the computer refused to obey my commands and you came to my rescue any time of the day or night.

In acknowledging my other thanks, the first name to spring to mind is that of Mrs Wendy Holton. Not only has she endlessly transported the discs back and forth, but her advice, suggestions and background knowledge have been unsurpassable. Her coffee has been welcome, too! I also have to thank her and her daughters Jennifer and Sarah for help with the Index.

Thanks are acknowledged to Fontana for permission to publish Figures 4, 12 and 28 from *Once a Month* (5th edn); to William Heinemann Medical Books to publish Figures 8, 9, 19, 20 and 41 from *The Premenstrual Syndrome and Progesterone Therapy* (2nd edn); to Oxford University Press to publish Figures 29 and 42 from *Depression After Childbirth* (2nd edn); to Peter Andrew Publishing to publish Figures 5 and 22 (by Tom Dalton) and 15, 16, 28 and 35 (by Glen Hutchinson) from *PMS Illustrated*; to W. B. Saunders and Co. for permission to include Figure 24 from S. S. C. Yen's and R. B. Jaffe's *Reproductive Endocrinology* (3rd edn). Thanks are also acknowledged to Chris Priest, who drew Figures 6, 7, 8, 9, 11, 12, 14, 23, 25, 26, 27, 29, 30, 44, 45 and 46.

KD
April 1994

INTRODUCTION:
DOES PMS EXIST?

The Professor of Human Metabolism at the University of London describes premenstrual syndrome (PMS) as the world's commonest disease, yet there is still no agreement among doctors about the best way to treat all sufferers. This is not surprising when one realizes that PMS comes in all shapes and sizes worldwide. There are over 150 different symptoms, it affects the teenager as well as her menopausal mother, the single parent and the single woman and embraces all social classes and ethnic groups. It is not only the woman who suffers; the greatest ordeal is sometimes inflicted on her partner, family, friends and workmates. But this should not be seen as a picture of doom and gloom – quite the reverse, with the wide range of 100 suggested treatments help is at the ready for all, however mild or however severe their suffering. Always remember that some treatments are advocated more for financial gain than purely to ease the suffering of the patient.

Of course, there are still quite a few people around, inside the medical profession and out, who continue to think that PMS is still 'a lot of nonsense', 'all in the mind', 'an excuse for weakness'. There is always establishment opposition to any new scientific theory or discovery. A famous scientist once stated that there never will be a case where all the opposers change their minds, they just gradually die and the new generation accepts the truth! In Physics, the two great advances this century were Einstein's theory of Relativity, and Quantum Mechanics. Einstein never did accept Quantum Mechanics (although he did much to make it possible); today it underlies all modern electronics, chemistry, biology and much more besides.

In the 1840s, a Hungarian physician called Ignaz Semmelweiss was bold enough to suggest that the awful number of mothers who died after childbirth from infections (then known as 'puerperal fever') might be lessened if doctors washed their hands before deliveries – in particular when they came direct from dissecting corpses in the mortuary! Although his method immediately turned out to be very effective in practice, and his junior colleagues were very quickly convinced, he was ridiculed by the senior people in his profession and actually driven out of his job. Tragically, he never did live to see his ideas universally accepted – this is often the case.

Nowadays practically all doctors and medical scientists accept that PMS exists, although it would be fair to say that there is still much disagreement about its causes and methods of treatment. There are still a few doctors around who tell PMS sufferers to 'pull themselves together' or who treat them for simple depression, but they become fewer each year. To quote from a very recent American book on the subject: 'Premenstrual Syndrome (PMS) has been a recognized clinical entity for many years . . . PMS is thought to be extremely prevalent.' (Samuel Smith and Isaac Schiff, *Modern Management of Premenstrual Syndrome*; New York and London: W. W. Norton & Co., 1993)

Apart from the inevitable Doubting Thomases, there are two major groups who still tend to disbelieve in PMS. One such group is to be found among psychologists: some psychologists still tend to believe that all mental disorders are caused by events in early life. This belief can no longer be held in quite such a pure form as in the days of Freud and Jung – there can no longer be any practising psychiatrists who refuse to accept the effectiveness of drugs in treating depression and schizophrenia, for example; nevertheless some are still inclined to give way as little as possible to what one might call the 'organic' (chemical) theory of psychiatry. As mental states and functions are more and more being shown to be governed by hormones, neurotransmitters and other chemicals, there is less room left for psychoanalysis as a treatment. (The authors of this book, on the other hand, tend to go to the other extreme and talk as if psychiatry will become obsolete in the near future when the endocrine system is fully understood. To be quite fair, this may also turn out to be a case of throwing the baby out with the bath water!) Please don't think that I am lumping all members of the psychiatric profession into this group; there are many who recognize the now obvious truth about PMS, with whom medical doctors can work. One of the patrons of the charity PMS Help is a very senior and distinguished psychiatrist. Still, there are quite a few of the other sort about.

The other major group of people who refuse to accept PMS is to be found among the more extreme feminists. As they see it, the existence of PMS means that women are not the equals of men; their political beliefs revolve around the article of faith that women are equal to men in all respects, and if anything conflicts with this belief then it must be wrong. Again, don't get the idea that I am claiming that all feminists think this way, but some, alas, do. Recently David Holton had a long interview with a woman journalist from one of our 'better' newspapers. The discussion covered a lot of ground, but at the end she managed to elicit the statement that some women with severe PMS, *if untreated*, would be disadvantaged for certain jobs. It was she who raised the topic. When the article appeared, the only point mentioned from the interview was that David Holton of PMS Help thought that women were no good for responsible jobs because they get PMS! I wonder how people like this journalist would explain the fact that in all physical sports there are separate classes for women. Women simply aren't generally as physically strong or powerful as men. Women have different skeletal proportions to men – they have narrower shoulders and larger hips, their forearms are shorter and overall they are shorter and lighter. These are facts, but they clearly do not mean that women are less valuable than men. We have to accept the world as it is; instead of bewailing or rationalizing away the fact of PMS, the authors of this book are trying to do something constructive about it; by freeing women from PMS we seek to remove this 'inequality' (if that is what it is). We would like to feel that we are doing more than some other (more politically motivated) people to help women.

In any case, the fact that all women experience menstruation does not mean that all women suffer from the *diseases* of menstruation. After all, we all have kidneys but we don't all have kidney disease. PMS is an illness, and one which does not affect all women.

I am often asked, 'if PMS is real, why has it only just recently been heard of?' It's a fair question, and the answer is:

a) It isn't new, but . . .
b) it certainly is a lot more common these days.

It is only in recent years that the subject of menstruation could ever be mentioned in public. It simply wasn't polite. Until 1970 the word was not allowed to be used in BBC broadcasts or in the newspapers. It therefore isn't surprising that PMS wasn't talked about, either. It probably wasn't even *thought* about by many 'respectable' people.

(Incidentally, as far as I know the first non-medical paper to use the word 'menstruation' in print was the *Radio Times*, when I was to give a talk on 'Schoolgirls and Menstruation' on BBC Radio 4's *Woman's Hour*. The editor wanted to change it to 'Schoolgirls and the Curse' or 'Schoolgirls and That Time of the Month'. When he finally agreed to use the dreadful word, it was spelled incorrectly!)

If one goes back in European literature to the centuries before the era of Victorian prudery – to the rumbustious literature of the 17th century, for example, or to Roman poets such as Ovid, one finds plenty of clear allusions to sex, but very few to menstruation. This is clearly one reason why PMS seems to us to be a recent phenomenon. There are not a lot of famous women in English history as traditionally taught – it's mostly about the doings of men – but reading between the lines one does sometimes dimly see behaviour in women which may well be explainable by PMS. Queen Victoria is a pretty clear example, but it's also worth reading about Queen Elizabeth I with PMS in mind; even if she did have 'the heart and stomach of a man', she presumably had the hormones of a woman. Elizabeth Barrett Browning and Catherine the Great of Russia might also be candidates for our suspicions. About the great mass of ordinary women in history we know practically nothing.

Of the three references to menstruation in the Bible, none seems to be about PMS, except just possibly Lamentations 1.15:

. . . the Lord hath commanded concerning Jacob, that his adversaries should be round about him: Jerusalem is as a menstruous woman among them.

This does seem to be using the words *menstruous woman* as a metaphor for particular weakness and helplessness.

Among the ancient Greeks, Hippocrates noted the symptoms of agitation and lethargy, which were clearly PMS, and which he attributed to the blood trying to escape from the body. (So once bleeding starts, the symptoms would naturally stop. This theory did explain the observed facts as he then knew them, and therefore was a good scientific theory. My theory is better because today there are more facts known, such as what tends to start PMS and what seems to cure it. My theory explains all of these, which Hippocrates' didn't and couldn't – and is therefore the better theory!).

As to part (b) of my reply: I am fairly sure that there is a lot more PMS around than ever before. In my view it is reaching almost epidemic proportions. I think that there are at least four clear reasons for this:

1. Fewer pregnancies
2. Stress
3. Diet
4. The contraceptive pill.

Before the advent of easy and reliable contraception, most women who married were pregnant for a very large fraction of their fertile lives. Nowadays, a woman might have 12 periods a year for, say, 35 years: that's 420 periods. If she has two children, she'll miss perhaps 25 to 30 of those periods (the minimum is 18, but don't forget breastfeeding). A century ago, she might well have had 12 children, (and many women had far more than 12), with prolonged breastfeeding used as a means of contraception, so that there were only one or two menstruations – if any – between pregnancies. She might have had only a tenth of the chances to feel PMS that the modern woman gets.

Does this sound far-fetched? It's a fact, and it happens now in under-developed countries – and even in Britain. I know of a woman with a large family who asked for help with her PMS when she was in her forties. When asked if she had suffered the symptoms when she was younger, she said that she couldn't remember – until recently she had not had a period since she was 18 years old!

As regards stress, remember that only recently have most women had jobs outside the home, let alone careers. Now, fortunately, they have (or should have!) equal opportunities in employment; but although this is in general an excellent development which I am unreservedly glad about, we all have to face the fact that today's women are under a lot more stress than ever before. After all, most working women have a home to run as well. Now, one of the things most authorities on PMS do agree about is that stress is a major contributory factor (see Chapter 4).

Today's women are also under immense pressure to be slim. This was not always so – just go to any art gallery and look at the women of previous centuries. Unless you believe that for many centuries all those painters were painting what they saw as undesirably plump women, you have to accept that the standard of beauty was different in those days. Poor old King Henry VIII – he agreed to marry his fourth wife, Anne of Cleves, on the strength of a painting, but when he saw her face to face he found her so ugly that the marriage was never consummated and he divorced her after six months. Her big trouble was that she was so slim! After the divorce she stayed at Henry's court, eating and drinking a lot; she soon put on weight and people said she had never looked so pretty! Going much further back in history: in the St Albans Museum there is a lovely, incredibly lifelike Roman statue of the goddess Venus – and she's pretty plump by 1990s standards, especially around the hips. If there is one figure who must have represented the Roman ideal of beauty, it's Venus, goddess of love.

But it wasn't only centuries ago that a degree of plumpness was considered beautiful – Marilyn Monroe was a size 16. Just look at any of those stars of the 1950s and 1960s. It's only in the last 20 years that extreme thinness has become so desirable.

To be as slim as the modern ideal, most women have to discipline themselves to eat much less than they might wish, and we shall see (in Chapter 6) that low blood sugar levels, caused by an inadequate diet, are by far the most important factor in causing PMS. Happily, this is also very easy to put right. We shall also see that it's the *timing* between meals or snacks that is particularly important – there must never be a gap of more than three hours (except when you're asleep). Just consider the traditional eating patterns of all but the poor, even up to quite recently: there would be a substantial breakfast, then a snack (remember *elevenses*?) before lunch. Between lunch and dinner people used to have tea, and there would also be supper, or some kind of snack before bed. If people kept to such a regime today we can be quite certain that there would only be about four PMS sufferers for every 10 who now exist – *and that would be true even if the meals were small enough to prevent women putting on undesirable weight!*

Don't forget that slimming is now a huge and profitable industry involving scores of publications, clubs, schemes and fashion and food products. Like some drug and health food industries it represents a vast and powerful block which is resistant to change from outside and, often, to simple and easy ideas from which there is no money to be made.

As for the Pill, I can only say that a huge number of women take it for at least part of their lives, and that I find in practice that starting or stopping the Pill is a common trigger for PMS. Again, it's a case of 'like it or lump it' – experience shows that it is so, whether we would wish it or not – but again, there are ways round it, as we shall see.

There it is, then. PMS *does* exist and it *does* affect a lot of women. The rest of this book will tell you more about the causes of PMS, and will review all the treatments, good or bad, which are commonly used today.

PART I

What Is PMS
and What Causes It?

Chapter 1

FREEDOM OF CHOICE

'Freedom of choice of medical treatment'. It sounds wonderful, but it is a privilege that is meaningless unless the sufferer understands the advantages and disadvantages of the many treatments available. In the search for relief of premenstrual syndrome (PMS) there is a bewilderingly wide variety of treatment options available. Everyone is free to choose what treatment they like, when they like and where they like. Women can select from treatments advertised in the media or over the counter; they can (in Britain) consult their NHS general practitioners (GPs) or get referred to consultants (be they gynaecologists, physicians, psychiatrists or endocrinologists). The choice extends to private medicine and alternative practitioners. Such a extensive selection does not make the choice any easier, rather the reverse. On the other hand, there may be limitations set by what the sufferer finds available locally, or by financial considerations.

The principal aim of this book is to lay out for you all the possible ways of relieving your PMS – and all the many and varied nostrums which are *claimed* to be of benefit, which is not necessarily the same thing! By the time you have read this book you should be in a position to choose for yourself the treatment(s) worth trying in your own case, and the end will be in sight! But first – are you suffering from PMS at all? Let's take a look at what PMS really is, and at some of the related conditions which fall within the scope of this book.

WHAT IS PMS?

PMS differs from all other diseases in that the diagnosis does not depend on the *type* of symptoms you suffer from, but solely on the time *when* your symptoms appear and disappear. The problems must begin within 14 days of the start of menstruation and there must always be at least seven clear symptom-free days after menstruation when normality returns.

> PMS is the presence of recurrent symptoms before menstruation with the complete absence of symptoms after menstruation.

We Are All Different

Already doctors have identified more than 150 different symptoms which can occur in PMS. Fortunately, no one has all of them! We are all different and have different symptoms, different combinations of symptoms and different timing of symptoms. We have different backgrounds, a different genetic make-up and different aspirations. We have our individual likes and dislikes, which affect our choice, so it is important to understand the host of different approaches.

WHAT IS A CURE?

I am convinced that out of every 10 women with real PMS-induced symptoms who read this book and faithfully carry out my main recommendations, five or six will gain enough relief to consider themselves completely 'cured', and another three or four will get a great deal of benefit. But what do we mean by the word 'cure'?

Let's consider a simple bacterial infection like tonsillitis. If you get it the doctor will give you antibiotics, the bacteria will die and you will probably be 'cured'. If the antibiotics don't completely get rid of the infection you may have to have your tonsils out; then you really will be cured. In that sense, a cure is something that gets rid of the problem and you don't have to worry about it any more. We can't cure PMS in that way, and we know enough about it to be fairly sure that we never shall.

We still don't have any satisfactory drug which will kill viruses in the way that antibiotics kill bacteria. Even with a mild and simple viral infection such as a cold, you just have to wait until your body builds up antibodies against the virus. You can go to bed and keep warm, which will give your body the best chance to fight back, but that's not *curing* your cold. When you take tablets to get rid of the headache which comes with the cold, or spray decongestants into your nose to unblock it, you are not killing the cold, just getting rid of the nastiest symptoms. This we call *symptomatic relief*, and many of the 'remedies' for PMS come under this heading. If they are all you need, then fine, you are lucky.

There is another type of illness – such as haemophilia, diabetes or hypothyroidism – which can be controlled by giving the patient some substance which he or she is lacking – factor 8 to the haemophiliac, insulin to the diabetic and thyroxine to the person with the underactive thyroid gland. This replacement therapy is not a cure, but it's more than just symptomatic relief. As long as the patient continues to receive treatment, the condition will be controlled, but treatment can never be stopped. PMS really falls into this group – there are ways of gaining symptomatic relief, which may be enough in mild cases, but to really get to the root of the trouble the patient is going to have to stick to a three-hourly carbohydrate diet (see Chapter 6) so that her body can make proper use of its own progesterone; she may possibly need to take extra progesterone as well. Unlike diabetics, however, PMS sufferers will only need treatment until the menopause, not for life.

Now many of these conditions are the sort that you can be born with, or born with a tendency to get. Haemophilia is an obvious example, so are heart disease and depression. People used to say that they 'run in families'. PMS is also known to run in families: daughters and sisters of PMS sufferers are more likely to be sufferers themselves. But in many or most cases of PMS there have certainly also been 'triggers' which start the PMS off – any hormonal upheaval, the changes brought on by puberty, childbirth or starting the Pill, can trigger off PMS in women who are already disposed to it.

So long as a PMS treatment makes a woman feel well, she probably doesn't care whether she's only gaining symptomatic relief or controlling the condition at its roots – but she must understand that she can never let up. If she stops taking whatever measures she finds effective, the PMS will be back. That's one of life's many unfairnesses.

HAVE YOU GOT PMS?

Before you decide what is likely to be the best approach to treatment for you, it is as well to be certain that your illness really is PMS and not some other problem which becomes worse as menstruation approaches. Sadly, one has to say that because there are a lot of different, conflicting views on PMS to be found in the medical profession, you can't be certain of getting the right treatment or even the right type of investigation. I don't mean that you're certain to get ineffective diagnosis and treatment – far from it, and the chances are fewer every year – but you may.

At the Hospital

In a hospital, of course, you will see a specialist for a long-term ailment like PMS; the relevant specialist in this case will be a gynaecologist.

Most gynaecologists rely on all sorts of physical tests to make a diagnosis – blood tests, hormonal estimations (tests for quantity), ultrasound scans, laparoscopies and abnormalities found when performing operations. All these gynaecological tests give normal results when done on a PMS sufferer (unless there is something else wrong with her) – the test we need is a way of estimating the number of progesterone receptors in the brain of sufferers and comparing them with the number in other women. (Unfortunately this test does not yet exist; the information which we do have about progesterone receptors comes from animal and post-mortem studies.)

Most medical scientists seem to think that if menstruation is stopped, the premenstruum (days before menstruation) with all its problems will stop, too. PMS sufferers who have had hysterectomies and no longer menstruate know that the solution is not quite as simple as that – the cyclical bouts of symptoms will keep on happening, even though the sufferer no longer menstruates. Only if menstruation has stopped in the natural way, after the menopause, will PMS go away of its own accord.

Consultant gynaecologists, in hospitals or elsewhere, rarely see a PMS patient many times, and so they tend not to realize that she has a long-term problem. On the first visit the patient will probably be seen by a consultant, then the next time she comes she is likely to be seen by the senior registrar (a more junior doctor). If she has benefited from the treatment, her own doctor (general practitioner) will be informed and advised to continue the treatment. If the patient has not responded to the treatment, another treatment will be tried and she will be given another appointment in two or three months' time, when she will often be seen by a more junior doctor.

If the second treatment is successful the patient will be discharged back to the general practitioner, but if she reports no benefit, yet another treatment will be tried and the next appointment will be timed so that she will be seen by a new junior doctor to follow up. In too many cases the consultant does not even realize that the woman is still attending the outpatient department. It follows from the above that many gynaecology departments are not going to have a lot of success with PMS.

General Practitioners

I nearly always see PMS patients *after* they have seen the GP, and I know from my considerable experience that GPs vary enormously in their approaches to PMS. I still hear far too often from patients that her GP doesn't believe PMS exists, and tells the woman to 'pull herself together'. Another favourite is: 'It'll go away when you have a baby.' (In fact it won't, and it might well get worse!) Others immediately reach for the prescription pad and issue antidepressants and/or tranquillizers – another dead end. (Incidentally, a PMS Help survey reveals that women doctors are not much better than men in this regard.)

Don't think I am judging these doctors too harshly. Some of them qualified 20 or 30 years ago, when PMS was unheard of. All doctors constantly have to keep up with the fantastically rapid advances being made by medical science in all areas. They do their best and cannot be blamed if they are a bit behind the times in one or two respects. Remember, too, that even today there are a lot of wrong ideas about PMS being given out by sincere and well-intentioned researchers; neither doctors nor patients can be blamed for being confused by all the conflicting information being bandied about.

I also encounter an awful lot of good GPs who take PMS seriously and who want to help but don't know how. Some frankly ask me, others don't know whom to ask; some think they know, but don't. Fortunately there are also some excellent general practitioners who realize that they themselves can easily treat PMS and who are ready to take a holistic approach and give the necessary time to discuss the patient's diet and personally monitor the effect of treatment.

So How Should It Be Diagnosed?

In PMS the symptoms or complaints only come before menstruation and disappear after menstruation. Furthermore, the complaints cannot start earlier than 14 days before menstruation and then tend to increase so that the worst time is immediately before the heavy bleeding starts (Figure 1). The same problems come each month at about the same phase in each menstrual cycle with monotonous regularity. Some women have slight bleeding for a day or more before the full menstrual flow, and they may find that their premenstrual problems are not eased until after the full bleeding.

Timing of PMS symptoms
- Never more than 14 days before menstruation
- Always at least 7 days without symptoms after menstruation

THE MENSTRUAL CHART

The way PMS is diagnosed is simplicity itself and can easily be done at home without any expensive blood tests, X-rays or even a physical examination. The easiest way, and the way most doctors will like you to approach the subject, is to draw up a 'menstrual chart' and write down daily the presence or absence of symptoms and of menstruation (Figure 2).

It is up to you to choose whichever symptoms you like to

1. The most common timing is the presence of symptoms commencing during the week before menstruation, with gradually increasing severity until menstruation commences.

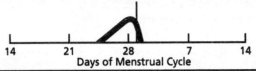

2. There may be short-lived symptoms at ovulation, easing for a few days, then recurring and increasing in severity to menstruation.

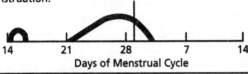

3. The symptoms may start at ovulation and continue with increasing severity until menstruation.

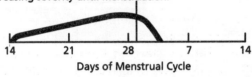

Figure 1: Severity of symptoms

record, but the process of daily recording is essential to a definitive diagnosis. Don't confuse the issue by writing down too many different symptoms, limit it to your *three* worst problems, and use a *single* letter to indicate each of the three symptoms. If you like, you can use a small letter for mild symptoms and a capital letter for serious symptoms. Or you may just like to mark with an 'x' the days when you feel awful, and an 'X' when it all becomes unbearable. What really matters is that the chart shows up the days of your periods and the days of your problems – this is how your doctor will be able to decide whether your problems are caused by PMS or not.

In the end each woman's chart will look quite different because some women will have symptoms for 10 or more days, others only a day or two before menstruation and for still others the symptoms might spill over into the start of menstruation itself (Figure 3).

It is quite normal for some women to have menstruation every 21 days, and others every 36 days. There may well be variations of three or four days between the lengths of your cycles, and yet

Name   Year **1994**

Day	Jan	Feb	Mar	Apr	May	Jun	Jul	Aug	Sep	Oct	Nov	Dec
1					M							M
2					M							M
3			x		M					x	x	M
4			x	X						X	x	
5			X	X						X	M	
6			X	M						M	M	
7			X	M						M	M	
8		M	Mx	M					x	M		
9		M		M					x	M		
10		X	M	M					X			
11		x							X			
12	x	X							M			
13	x	M					x		M			
14	X	M						X	M			
15	X	M					X	X	M			
16	M	M					x	X	M			
17	M						X	M				
18	M						M	Mx				
19						x	M	M				
20						x	M	M				x
21					x	x						X
22					x	x						X
23					x	X						X
24					X	M						M
25					X	M						M
26					M	M						M
27					M							M
28				x	M						x	
29				x	M						x	
30				X							x	
31												

Figure 2: Simple menstrual chart (M = menstruation;
x = mild symptoms; X = severe symptoms)

doctors would consider the menstruation perfectly regular.

What is a normal menstrual pattern?
- Loss lasting between 2 and 8 days
- Length of cycle between 21 and 36 days
- Length of cycle varying by up to 4 days each month

Keep the chart up regularly as you try out different treatments, so that you have a visual record of the success or otherwise of different approaches.

Despite these individual variations, the cyclical nature of PMS stands out very clearly on a chart. The best way is to stand back

Name   Year

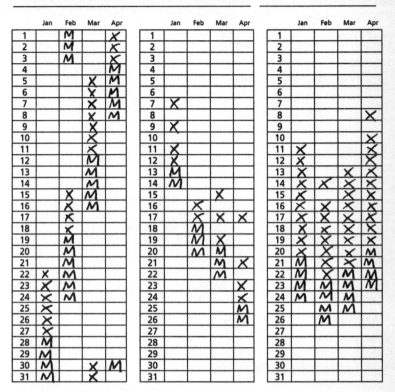

Figure 3: Three menstrual charts showing different menstrual cycles and timing of symptoms (M = menstruation; X = symptoms)

from it. Don't focus on the letters, but look at the pattern. Of all the hundreds of slides I use in lectures, one of my favourites shows some menstrual charts in Japanese! (Figure 4.) I can't read a word of it, but the fact that the women suffer from PMS is as plain as a pikestaff.

It is no good guessing that you have a 28-day cycle, as 28 days is only the average length – only charting will tell you accurately. There is a story that long ago there was a mid-European country where a woman could claim the title of 'Menstrual Princess' and claim a state pension if her cycle was always exactly 28 days. Certainly, in Britain today there would be very few, if any, women able to make this claim (apart from those who take the Pill).

	1月	2月	3月	4月	5月	6月	7月	8月	9月	10月	11月	12月
1						月						
2						月						
3									セ			
4									セ			
5									セ			
6									セ			
7									セ			
8				キ				ズ	月・セ			
9				キ				ズ	月・セ			
10		キ		キ				ズ	月	セ		
11		キ		月・キ				ズ		セ		
12		キ	キ	月・キ				ズ		セ		
13		キ	キ	月			月・ズ			月・セ		
14		キ	月・キ	月			月・ズ			月		
15		キ	月	月			月・ズ			月	セ	
16	キ・セ	月・キ	月	月						月	セ	
17	キ	月	月				ズ	月		月	セ	セ
18	キ	月					ズ	月			セ	セ
19	月・キ						月・ズ	月			月・セ	セ
20	月						月・ズ				月	セ
21	月						月・ズ				月	セ
22	月							月			月	セ
23						ズ		月			月	月・セ
24						月・ズ		月				月・セ
25						月・ズ		月				月
26					ズ	月・ズ						月
27					ズ	月						
28					ズ	月						
29					月・ズ	月・ズ						
30					月	月						
31					月							
計												

月：月経　ズ：頭痛　キ：緊張　セ：背中の痛み

Figure 4: Japanese menstrual charts showing PMS

Look at the typical chart showing PMS (Figure 2). Don't expect the characteristic PMS pattern to run horizontally across the chart like a bar. First, we have already noted that very few women (if any) have a precisely regular 28-day cycle. Secondly, each column has 31 boxes and five of the 12 months don't have 31 days. Lastly, a woman's PMS symptoms don't always start on precisely the same day of her cycle. For these reasons the marks in the columns on the chart don't line up exactly opposite last month's marks, but are offset a little, usually upwards. Thus, when viewed at a distance, the chart tends to show a diagonal bar, usually sloping up to the right if the cycle is shorter than 30 days, or down to the right if it is longer than 31 days.

THE CHARACTERISTICS OF PMS

The diagnosis of PMS depends entirely on the timing of the symptoms in relation to menstruation. If the cyclical pattern is there, then it's PMS, whatever the symptoms. If the pattern is *not* there, then it's not PMS. Even so, there are certain characteristics which would suggest to a doctor that a woman is prone to the disease and which tend to be pointers to those patients most at risk.

PMS starts at times of hormonal change or upheaval, such as:
- puberty (accompanying the onset of menstruation)
- after pregnancy, especially if complicated by pre-eclampsia or postnatal depression
- after using the Pill
- when menstruation starts again after missing more than three months
- after sterilization
- after removal of an ovary.

Doctors are becoming increasingly aware that PMS often starts as early as when periods first begin. Too many girls are classed as 'awkward adolescents' when it is really their hormones that are being awkward. This includes those bright girls who suddenly deteriorate in their behaviour and/or school work between the ages of 12 and 15 years. Teachers know only too well what I mean. All too often the girls themselves cannot understand what has happened to them, or why the world has suddenly turned sour. It is the teachers who should be alert to the possibility of PMS in this age group (and, of course, should know how to refer these girls to someone for advice).

Another time when PMS often starts is after a pregnancy, when it's all too easy to blame the woman's changed character and mood swings on the difficulty of handling the extra responsibility of motherhood. In such cases it is the midwife or health visitor who should be on the lookout for PMS and able to advise the patient where to get treatment.

Then again, development of PMS when one is on the Pill is very gradual and therefore easy to miss, so it is often only when

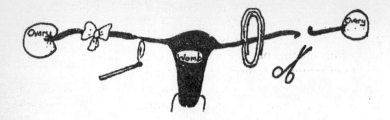

Figure 5: Sterilization increases PMS whether the tubes are tied, cut, clipped or cauterized

the Pill is stopped that the on/off pattern of irritability is recognized. These sufferers are frequently seen at Family Planning Clinics where they so often go for help.

Sterilization is another common starting-point for PMS. It doesn't matter if the sterilization is done by cutting, clipping, cautery or stitching – in all cases PMS may start afterwards, and PMS will not improve if the tubes are joined together again, even if it is done so successfully that a pregnancy results (Figure 5).

Even if the symptoms of PMS started mildly at puberty, they are likely to get worse at the other times just mentioned, such as after a pregnancy, after a spell of amenorrhoea (missing periods), or after the Pill or the removal of an ovary.

Most PMS sufferers have difficulty in tolerating the Pill because they develop depression, headaches, gain in weight, nausea or bloatedness. They are the ones who tend to try several brands and then finally settle for a different, non-hormonal method of contraception. This is not surprising, because all oral contraceptives contain *progestogens*, the man-made drugs which lower the blood progesterone level (see Chapter 4).

Many PMS sufferers have difficulty in coping with alcohol, especially red wine. In the 'good' times they can have their daily tipple without any problem, but then during their final premenstrual days they may find that they become intoxicated by an amount which would normally not bother them. What is worse, they tend to have a great urge for more alcohol at these times, and may find that they regularly exceed the advised limit once a month.

Although they do not necessarily include it in their list of symptoms, a very high proportion of PMS sufferers have difficulty in controlling their occasional binges and cravings, usually for chocolates, sweets, starchy or even salty foods. The full reason for this phenomenon is given in Chapter 4, and the way to overcome it is discussed in Chapter 6.

A five-pound weight swing twice a month at ovulation and menstruation is quite normal and healthy, and is not necessarily a sign of PMS. But what is significant is when there is a weight swing in either direction of two stone or more at any time during adult life. Think of your lowest ever weight since the age of 16 years, and subtract it from your highest ever (non-pregnant) weight. If the difference is over two stone, then that tends to suggest that you are at risk of developing or having PMS.

Young teenagers (and adult women as well) may find they have an increased sex urge premenstrually. This *nymphomania* was recognized by an American, Dr S. I. Israel, as long ago as 1938.

There is a tendency for PMS to run in families. In the author's practice, several examples have been recorded of PMS running through three generations, each diagnosis being confirmed by menstrual charts and each having been treated for PMS. Studies undertaken in Finland, Australia and London have all confirmed the very high incidence of PMS in identical twins, who have the same genetic make-up, compared with a much lower incidence of PMS in pairs of non-identical twins, who would have only half the same genetic component. The incidence of PMS in non-identical twins is nearer that found in sisters, who also would have only half of the same genetic components. Another London survey of adopted daughters suffering from PMS found that their adoptive mothers, who would have had a completely different genetic composition, had a low incidence of PMS, compared with higher incidence of PMS in biological mothers, whose PMS daughters would have had half the same genetic components. John Condon, who studied 300 volunteer twin pairs from the Australian National Health and Medical Research Council Twin Registry, concluded that environmental effects did not have much influence on the incidence of PMS, which was overwhelmingly due to the genetic factor, although the precise gene has not yet been isolated.

> ## Common characteristics of PMS and its sufferers
> - PMS starts at time of hormonal event
> - PMS increases in severity at time of hormonal event
> - Sufferers experience side-effects while on the Pill
> - Difficulty tolerating alcohol
> - Tendency to food cravings and binges
> - Adult weight swing exceeds two stone
> - Increased sex urge
> - Mother also suffers (or suffered) PMS

PMS IS A CHRONIC DISEASE

Once you have PMS you are likely to continue having it until the menopause, but that does not mean that it will always be as severe. There will be months or years when it fades into the background, is not so important and doesn't rule your life. There will be other times when it can cause chaos. Perhaps the biggest factor which increases the severity of PMS is stress, which is something none of us can avoid altogether and which can involve our life at home, work or play (see list below).

Stress is not something new, not something to do only with life in modern times, although writers on the subject often tend to give that impression. If you read newspapers from earlier this century you will notice that even then stress featured quite a lot (though not then known by that name), and that writers then attributed problems to the speed of life brought about by trains, electricity, telephones and so on. It was Hans Selye, the Nobel prize-winner, who introduced the word 'stress' and by a series of ingenious experiments on rabbits showed that stress caused hormonal effects on the adrenal glands, causing a release of cortisone.

> ## Factors which cause PMS to increase in severity
> - Stress
> - Large weight gain or loss
> - Night work
> - Alcohol
> - Smoking

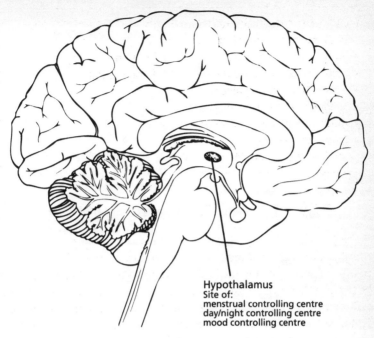

Hypothalamus
Site of:
menstrual controlling centre
day/night controlling centre
mood controlling centre

Figure 6: Controlling centres of the brain

A woman's PMS may have been well controlled until for some unrelated reason there is a sudden weight increase or weight loss. This may coincide with a complete change of environment, such as being at university, spending a year 'nannying' in Italy or travelling round the world. These are times when life is so interesting that you tend to forget about food, and either overeat or miss meals. Rigid dieting is another very common factor; the more successful you are at dieting, the greater the chance of increasing your PMS. Life can be so unfair!

The *hypothalamus* in the lower part of the brain houses most of the body's controlling centres, including the centres controlling menstruation and pregnancy, weight maintenance and day/night rhythm (Figure 6).

This explains why PMS is affected by marked weight changes, and also why PMS is so often aggravated by night work and long-distance flights. Some will say that PMS affects all the pleasures of life, for it does become worse when tasting enjoyable night life, with alcohol and with smoking!

17

Chapter 2

IF IT'S NOT PMS

PMS has been described as 'one of the few diseases that is persistently being investigated in patients that do *NOT* have the disease'. So when you've kept your chart for two or more months, don't be too disheartened if you are told you do not suffer from PMS. Even if it is some other illness, it is still worthwhile considering the other causes for your symptoms so that you can receive the appropriate treatment. How often does one hear the distraught woman say 'but it must be PMS! I have these terrible mood swings . . . bloatedness . . . breast tenderness . . . times when I want to end it all.' But none of these symptoms in itself adds up to PMS – after all, they can all occur in men and non-menstruating women. The only thing that makes them PMS is their regular appearance and disappearance with the stages of your menstrual cycle.

There are some menstrual problems, which, when carefully recorded, turn out not to be PMS. In fact most medical PMS Clinics in Britain, the US and throughout the world will tell you that about half of all women who attend do not have PMS but suffer from some other menstrual problem. Among the common ailments masquerading as PMS are *menstrual distress, dysmenorrhoea, endometriosis, postnatal depression* and the *menopause*. In the following chapters these conditions will be considered as I discuss the values of the various treatments.

MENSTRUAL DISTRESS

This is when your symptoms are present throughout the cycle but get worse during the premenstruum (the days before the

Chart 1

Day	Jan	Feb	Mar	Apr
1				X
2				
3		X		
4		X		
5		X		
6			X	
7				
8	X			
9	X			
10	X		X	
11	X		X	
12	X		X	
13		X		
14		X		X
15		X		X
16				X
17			X	
18	X		X	
19	X		X	
20	X			
21	X	M		
22		M		M
23	M	M	M	M
24	M	M	M	M
25	M	M	M	M
26	M	M	M	M
27	M	M	M	M
28	M		M	
29			X	
30			X	
31	X			

Chart 2

Day	Jan	Feb	Mar	Apr
1				
2				
3			X	
4				
5	X			
6				
7				
8				
9				
10				
11				
12	X			
13		X		
14	M			
15	M			
16	M			
17	X			
18				
19				
20		M		
21		M		X
22		M		
23				
24	X		X	
25				
26				
27				
28			M	
29			M	
30			M	M
31				M

Chart 3

Day	Jan	Feb	Mar	Apr
1		M	M	MX
2	X	M	MX	M
3	X	M		
4		M		
5	X	X		
6			X	
7	M	X		
8	MX	X		X
9	M			X
10	M			
11				
12	X			
13			X	X
14				X
15				X
16		X		
17		X		
18		X		
19			X	
20	X		X	
21			X	
22				
23				X
24	X	X		M
25				M
26		M	X	M
27	X	M		M
28	X	M		X
29			X	
30			M	
31			M	X

Figure 7: Charts showing menstrual distress (M = menstruation; X = symptoms)

period) or at the time of menstruation. Sometimes the symptoms are present every day of the month, or they may only be occurring occasionally – sometimes during the postmenstruum (the days after the period is over) but more frequently before or during menstruation. Menstrual distress – or *menstrual magnification* as the Americans would prefer to call it – is the commonest problem found in women who attend PMS Clinics but who turn out not to have PMS (Figure 7).

It is always difficult to decide whether to give PMS treatment to those with menstrual distress. They should never be included as volunteers for clinical trials of PMS, and should be aware that PMS is not their only problem. The usual consensus is that women with only mild or occasional symptoms during the postmenstruum will benefit most from PMS treatment, even

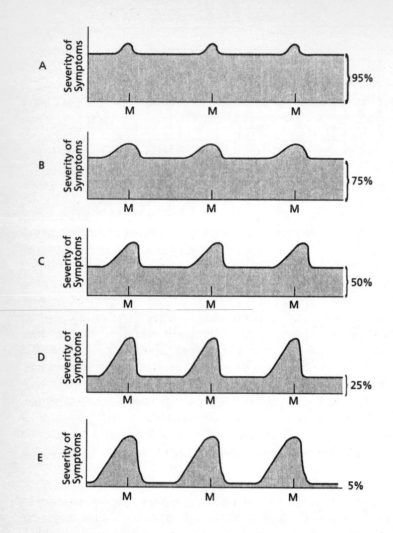

Figure 8: Varying severity of PMS exacerbation in menstrual distress

though their problems after menstruation will remain. However, those who have serious symptoms throughout the cycle, with a relatively small increase in symptoms before their period and possibly during the first day or two of the period, are likely to respond better to treatment for their underlying disease (Figure 8).

DYSMENORRHOEA

Dysmenorrhoea simply means 'painful menstruation'. It may be either *primary* (occurring from puberty onwards) or *secondary* (occurring some years after the time menstruation and ovulation are well established). Primary dysmenorrhoea is of two very different types, *spasmodic* or *congestive*.

Primary Dysmenorrhoea

Spasmodic Dysmenorrhoea

This usually comes on a year or two after menstruation has started at puberty, and only if ovulation (egg production) is occurring. (Nearly all girls' first few periods are *anovular* – no egg is produced.) There are no warnings during the premenstruum, but the spasms of pain occur with the start of bleeding (Figure 9). The spasms come about every 20 minutes, causing the girl to bend over or roll up in pain, being happiest lying rolled up with a hot-water bottle on her lower abdomen. The pain may spread to the back and inner sides of her thighs, and there may be reflex vomiting or fainting. She is likely to look pale, or even green, and may have beads of sweat on her forehead. The severe pain usually only lasts for one day, but there are some sufferers for whom some milder pain lasts into the next day or two. The pain eases gradually over the next 10 years and has usually disappeared by the time the sufferer is in her mid-twenties. It also usually disappears after a full-term pregnancy.

Congestive Dysmenorrhoea

This is one of the symptoms of PMS. The dysmenorrhoea may start with the first menstruation and continues regularly thereafter with each period. The woman has a dull, aching, continuous pain and bloatedness in her lower abdomen during the previous week or two, gradually becoming worse until the first day of menstruation, when it is at its height, and then it subsides (Figure 10). The pain is usually accompanied by some of the 'misery symptoms' of PMS, such as mood swings, irritability, tiredness, headaches or breast tenderness.

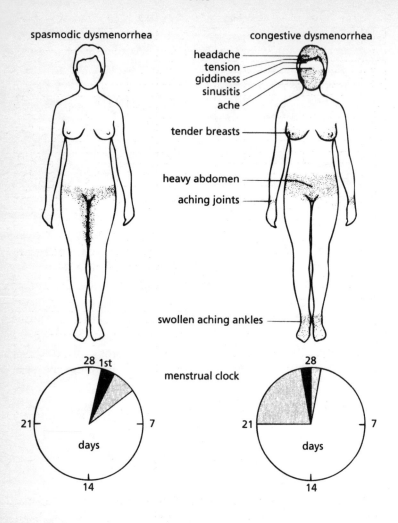

spasmodic dysmenorrhea

congestive dysmenorrhea

headache
tension
giddiness
sinusitis
ache

tender breasts

heavy abdomen

aching joints

swollen aching ankles

menstrual clock

Figure 9: Site and time of pain in spasmodic and congestive dysmenorrhoea

Secondary Dysmenorrhoea

As I said above, this means painful periods which begin later in life. It is always due to some other medical condition such as an infection (pelvic inflammatory disease) or adhesions, and needs professional medical treatment.

Spasmodic

Day	Jan	Feb	Mar	Apr	May
1					
2					
3					
4					
5					
6					
7					
8					
9					
10					
11					
12					
13					
14					MX
15					MX
16	XM			MX	M
17	XM			MX	M
18	M	MX	Mx	M	M
19	M	M	MX	M	
20	M	M	M	M	
21		M	M		
22			M		
23					
24					
25					
26					
27					
28					
29					
30					
31					

Congestive

Day	Jan	Feb	Mar	Apr	May
1					
2					
3					
4					
5				X	
6				X	X
7		X		X	X
8		X	X	X	X
9	X	X	X	X	X
10	X	X	X	X	X
11	X	X	X	X	X
12	X	X	X	X	XM
13	X	X	X	X	M
14	X	X	X	XM	M
15	X	X	X	M	M
16	X	X	X	M	M
17	X	X	XM	M	M
18	X	XM	M	M	
19	X	M	M	M	
20	MX	M	M	M	
21	M	M	M		
22	M	M	M		
23	M	M			
24	M				
25					
26					
27					
28					
29					
30					
31					

Figure 10: Charts of sufferers of spasmodic and congestive dymenorrhoea (M = menstruation; X = pain)

ENDOMETRIOSIS

This can also start with the first period or after years of normal menstruation. It causes pain before and throughout menstruation and is accompanied by painful intercourse, pain on moving the uterus when the doctor examines the patient, and infertility. The cells which form the lining of the cavity of the uterus (womb), and are normally shed through the vagina at each menstruation, are called 'endometrial' cells. Sometimes these endometrial cells find their way into other parts of the body, such as within the muscle wall of the womb or anywhere in the pelvis near the Fallopian tubes, ovaries, bladder or rectum. When menstruation occurs, these endometrial cells cannot be

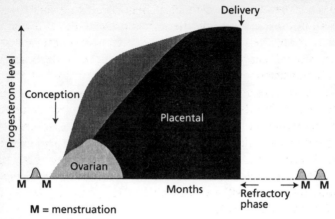

Figure 11: Blood progesterone levels in a normal menstrual cycle, during pregnancy and after giving birth (puerperium)

shed like normal cells through the vagina, but instead form cysts which gradually expand with each menstruation, causing increasing pain. This is because the wrongly placed endometrial cells still receive the messenger hormones telling them that menstruation has begun but, being in the wrong place, they don't have a way out.

Endometriosis needs expert medical help and is not suitable for self-help remedies or over-the-counter treatments. If you think you are suffering from endometriosis, go straight to Chapter 11.

POSTNATAL DEPRESSION

In a way, postnatal depression (PND) is the same thing as PMS, because it is caused by a sudden drop in the level of progesterone in the blood. During pregnancy this level rises enormously as the placenta produces up to 40 times the usual amount of progesterone (see Figure 11). This is why PMS sufferers often feel so well during pregnancy. When the child is born, the placenta is shed and the level of progesterone in the blood drops like a stone. The result may be just the slight 'baby blues' which nearly all mothers experience, but at the other end of the scale the mother may become insane and even kill her baby.

If we define postnatal depression as psychiatric symptoms

severe enough to require medical help, occurring for the first time in mothers after childbirth and before the return of normal menstruation, then one finds a close relationship between PMS and postnatal depression. As long ago as 1855 Dr Marce, a French physician, noted that women in his wards who were suffering from puerperal psychosis improved after each menstruation but then had a recurrence of symptoms before the next menstruation. In fact one study following up women who had previously suffered from postnatal depression showed that some 80 per cent of the subjects subsequently suffered from PMS. It is therefore not surprising that some treatments recommended for PMS are also valuable for postnatal depression (see Chapters 6 and 10).

Having said this, there are some other causes of mental illness after childbirth. For example, previous problems with manic depression or schizophrenia may return, or an illness may even start after the birth. It is for this reason that expert evidence must be available to the courts in cases such as infanticide, when PND is claimed as a defence.

THE MENOPAUSE

PMS tends to increase in severity when women reach their forties, possibly after pregnancies, after stopping the Pill or after a sterilization, and those women who find the symptoms severe enough to require treatment at this time are as likely as not to blame it all on the menopause, about which they have read so much. However PMS and the menopause are two quite different conditions and require quite different treatments. The menopause is a natural physiological state marking the shutdown of the reproductive apparatus and the end of childbearing. The usual age of the menopause, or the last menstruation, is between 45 and 55 years. The menopause is characterized by hot flushes and night sweats; dryness of the vagina, which causes painful intercourse; frequency of passing water; thinning of the layer of fat under the skin, so that wrinkles and crowsfeet appear; generalized joint pains and possibly the psychological symptoms of depression, anxiety and forgetfulness (Figure 12).

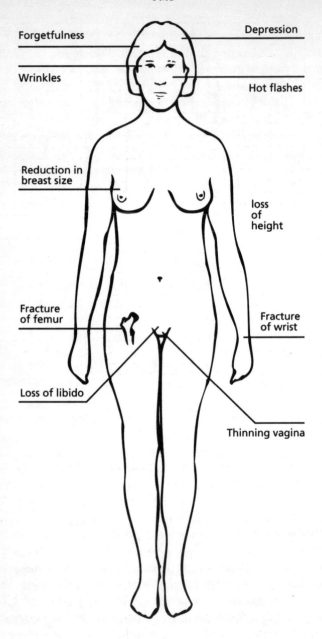

Figure 12: Sites of menopausal symptoms

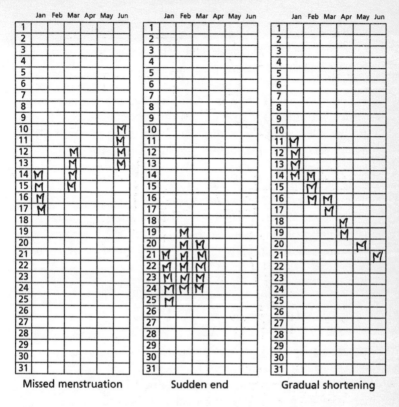

Figure 13: Menstrual charts of women at the menopause

These symptoms are continuous and do not come and go with each menstruation, as PMS does. At the menopause, menstruation gradually becomes infrequent and/or scanty, and ovulation ceases (Figure 13).

At the menopause the ovaries stop producing oestrogen. When the oestrogen level drops, the pituitary gland starts producing a lot more follicle stimulating hormone (FSH) as a sort of signal to the ovaries, trying to force them to take action and produce more oestrogen. It is possible to measure the level of FSH in the blood, which means that there is a simple blood test for the menopause. If the menopause has arrived, the level of FSH in the blood will be raised above the normal level found during the menstruating years.

27

Don't just guess!
At the Menopause the FSH level is raised.

This is an important test, as one finds women in their late thirties or forties blaming all their woes on the menopause, and hoping to get relief by being given hormone replacement therapy (HRT) (see page 137) – but if they aren't going through the menopause, the HRT would be too early and would give no benefit. The average age of the menopause is 50 years.

After the menopause the oestrogen which a woman's body needs is made in her peripheral cells and should maintain her bones in good condition. If there is not sufficient oestrogen after the menopause, she may develop osteoporosis (brittle bone disease).

OTHER SYMPTOMS

There are also many instances when you feel your symptoms are related to menstruation but your chart does not confirm this. It is not PMS, but what is it? The symptoms must have been those which come and go, so let's consider some other reasons for the attacks. It's time to consider the *when?*, the *how?*, the *why?* and the *what?*

We are all different and our problems are all different, but it is well worthwhile giving further thought to your symptoms before you go out to look for help. The more information you give to your doctor or health practitioner about your symptoms, the more chance the diagnosis will be the correct one.

When?
Having decided that your problem does not always come before menstruation or on a particular day of the week, see what time of the day it starts, how long it lasts and if it gets better in the evening. Try and decide what starts the symptom. There are countless possibilities. It might be worse (or better) after a lazy day in the sun, after a visit to the theatre or to your mother-in-law, or when there's an exam, interview or premiere coming up.

Is it worse in the winter or summer? If each year it seems to start up in October and then to improve by April, could it be *Seasonal Affective Disorder*, better known as *SAD*? If so, the future looks bright for you, as we now understand the importance of light and can cure SAD simply by exposing the patient to bright light for a few hours each day.

SAD is caused by hormones in the skin which need stimulating by light, so when the dark evenings appear and we cover up our skin with woollies, this light stimulation is lost. If this is a possibility for you, there is help available. Get in touch with SAD (their address is given in the Useful Addresses section).

How?

Give some thought to how an attack starts, how it progresses and how it ends. For instance, some headaches start with flashes of light, zigzags in front of the eyes, numbness or pins and needles down one side of the body. These are called 'aura', and occur in *Classical Migraine*. Some headaches seem to come with a cold, and then carry on, and are worse when you bend down – this would suggest *Sinusitis*. Other headaches start at the back of the head and spread down the neck to the shoulders – this is characteristic of a *Tension Headache*, which tends to come at times of stress.

Why?

There is always a reason for the attacks, although we may not always be able to put a finger on it. Nevertheless, it's worth giving a thought to why they should appear on, say, Monday and not on Thursday (or whatever day it might be). This is called searching for the 'trigger' which sets off the trouble. The trigger may not have occurred immediately before the start of the attack – often it will be about 24 hours earlier. This is particularly so with certain foods, which can cause a migraine or asthma attack. If necessary, use an attack form (see next page) and note down all that has occurred and all the food and drink consumed during the 24 hours immediately before the start of the attack. Do not then try to analyse the form immediately, but wait until you have three or more, then compare them carefully. You may find that the same item of food was involved every time, for instance onions, cheese or red wine. Or you may find that the attack comes after you've missed a meal, had a late night or eaten a Chinese meal.

Table 1: Attack Form

ATTACK FORM

Day and Date ....Type of Attack ....

Time of starting ....How long did it last? ....

During the **24 hours before** the attack
1.   Did you have any special worry, overwork or shock?
2.   What had you done during the day? Normal work? Unusual activity? Extra tired?

Please draw a line across the page when your attack started, then list everything you ate and drank during the **24 hours before** its start. The information above the line will be what you ate on that day; below the line, on the day before.

Breakfast..Time......................
....

Mid-morning ....Time......................
....

Lunch ....Time......................
....

Mid-afternoon ....Time......................
....

Supper...Time......................
....

Evening ....Time......................
....

Time of waking ....Time of going to bed...................

What do you think caused this attack?

What?

As with the when? it is useful to know what sparks off an attack. Again, the possibilities are innumerable, for we all lead such different lives, but it is worthwhile spending some time and thought on what might be triggering your trouble. Is it seeing certain individuals, your director or headteacher, your ex-partner or in-law? Are the symptoms likely to come on before or after certain activities, such as before examinations or while waiting for results? At weddings, christenings or funerals? Before or after shopping expeditions? Are they worse before, during or after holidays, or do they disappear entirely when you are away from home? If you find a possible cause but don't know what to do about it, discuss the problem with family, friends, a counsellor or a doctor. Try to take some constructive action to avoid the trigger causing chaos in future.

Healthy and Unhealthy Symptoms

It is easy to forget that the main symptoms of *premenstrual tension* (PMT) – tiredness, depression, aggression and irritability – can all occur in a perfectly healthy individual.

Tiredness

Watch the athletes on TV after they've run their 1,500 or 10,000 metres. They are all absolutely exhausted (of course), yet they are in tip-top health. So when you feel dead tired after a day's grind in the office and finish up with a swim, tennis or whatever, don't be alarmed if you, too, feel exhausted. I recall a young American woman in her early twenties who was so tired that she would fall asleep for about an hour after her midday snack. When medically examined she was healthy and all her blood tests were normal. When the doctor discussed her day's routine, it turned out that she got up at five each morning to jog round Regent's Park for an hour before breakfast, then took a quick shower and dashed off to work – pushing the tea trolley round a massive office. Hers was healthy and normal tiredness, there was no cause for alarm.

Depression

This can be a normal emotion as well as being a disease state. If

31

your nearest and dearest is involved in an accident, if your neighbour's house goes up in flames or your beloved dog dies, it is natural to be upset. In fact, if at such times you are not affected emotionally and the unexpected disaster does not appear to sadden you, it would actually be abnormal. Tears are perfectly normal in such situations.

Aggression
In moderation this symptom is important to most women, who will never reach the top without the necessary determination. However, there is a world of difference between useful aggression and PMS-type aggression and rages.

Irritability
This falls in the same category as aggression. If you are handed the wrong change in a shop, are falsely accused, have someone else use your credit card or find your holiday plane has been overbooked, you have every right to be irritable and annoyed. If you weren't, and remained emotionally flat, that would be abnormal. Again, however, these natural reactions are quite different from the intense irritability that can be a symptom of PMS.

Common Causes of Other Symptoms

It was stressed at the beginning of this chapter that all the possible PMS symptoms can also occur in men, children and postmenopausal women. But all 150 symptoms can also be due to some other cause, so it's worth considering some of the alternative causes of these symptoms.

Tiredness
This is often associated with *anaemia,* in which case it is worth thinking about your diet. Does it contain plenty of fruit, fresh vegetables and iron-rich foods? Or are you having heavy periods and losing blood faster than you can make it up from your food? This can also happen slowly with bleeding gums or piles. *Low thyroid function* is another common cause of tiredness, dullness and depression, and is accompanied by general coldness, dry skin and weight gain.

Anxiety
Anxiety can occur in patients with an overactive thyroid, in which case it may also be accompanied by a hearty appetite, tiredness, loss of weight and tremor. This is a condition which responds well to medical treatment, and which should be treated early in case it affects the heart.

Breast Tenderness
There are many causes of breast tenderness besides PMS. It is as well to remember that the breasts are sex organs, and many women find that breast tenderness or pain will fluctuate with their love life. If there is any leakage from the breasts, or if any lumps are felt, then an early medical examination is essential. Don't waste time with self-help measures or alternative medicines. Sensitivity of the nipples or areas of numbness on the breast may be a sign of *pyridoxine overdose neuropathy*, which generally eases as soon as vitamin B_6 (pyridoxine) is stopped (see Chapter 8).

Asthma/Rhinitis
The most frequent cause of asthma and rhinitis is an allergy, but finding what you are allergic to, and preventing contact with it, is often difficult. It may be pollens, moulds, fungi, dust, dust mites, cats, dogs, horses, specific foods, drugs or 101 other items. It gets worse with recurrent coughs and colds and with smoking.

Bone or Joint Pains
If this is the problem it is worth thinking about the when?, how?, why? and what? before seeking help. Does it follow the first game of sport in the season? If so, continue with the sport, but not quite so vigorously until your muscles are really up to scratch. Did it start after a fall, or after you'd done some strenuous decorating or hill-climbing? It is worth knowing which joints suffered first and which only later on. Is there any stiffness, and if so, when? Is it in the morning, and how long does it last? If the joint is hot or swollen, then seek advice early and blood tests will sort out the important problems from the mild ones that will disappear without treatment.

Nausea and Abdominal Pain

Recurrent attacks may be caused by food or drink – not necessarily the last food that was eaten, but possibly something you had a day or two before. If other members of the family or friends suffer at the same time, it is likely to be caused by food. *Irritable bowel syndrome* is often blamed on PMS, but only careful charting will distinguish it.

Colds

Coughs, colds and sore throats may keep recurring in persons with low resistance. They are particularly likely to occur in households with young schoolchildren, where the offending organism is originally caught at school but is then passed round from one member of the family to the others. After a time, bacteria lose their sensitivity to a given antibiotic and the antibiotic must be changed.

Chapter 3

WHAT DOES IT FEEL LIKE?

The magic figure of 'over 150 symptoms' is usually quoted by doctors to emphasize the great variety of complaints which may be covered by PMS. For those who only think in terms of 'Premenstrual Tension' (PMT), it is as well to appreciate that more than two thirds of all symptoms are physical, affecting some other part of the body, rather than psychological, or 'all in the mind' (Figure 14).

Fortunately, no one woman suffers from all the possible symptoms, although in the typical case doctors expect to find that there is more than one symptom – usually about five or six.

Psychological symptoms are the most common, and include:

- Tension
- Depression
- Irritability
- Lethargy
- Mood swings
- Irrationality
- Impatience
- Indecisiveness
- Inability to concentrate
- No sense of humour
- Paranoia
- Pessimism
- Anxiety
- Aggression
- Self-mutilation.

Among the more common bodily symptoms are:

- Bloatedness

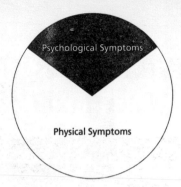

Figure 14: Proportion of physical and psychological PMS symptoms

• Breast tenderness
• Backache
• Bingeing
• Headache
• Migraine
• Nausea and vomiting
• Asthma
• Hay fever
• Sore throat
• Flu-like sensations
• Aching joints
• Pimples
• Cystitis
• Conjunctivitis

Doctors have also recorded the occurrence of some rare and obscure diseases which have been found to occur only in the premenstruum, with normality returning after menstruation, but we will not need to discuss these rarities here.

It is not only the psychiatrist who sees patients with PMS; every medical speciality gets involved at one time or another, including the neurologist, dermatologist, rheumatologist, ophthalmologist, allergist, urologist, otologist, dental surgeon, chest and cardiac physicians. (Don't worry what all these 'ologists' do – it doesn't matter. The point is that the poor patient gets sent from pillar to post.)

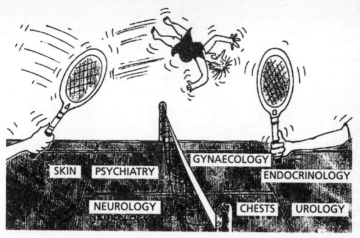

Figure 15: PMS sufferers go from specialist to specialist

No two women have the same combination of symptoms or the same order of priority of their problems. With such a huge range of individual symptoms, and appreciating that each woman has several combinations of them, one hardly needs to emphasize that each patient requires individual consideration of what the best method of treatment is for her. The problem each PMS sufferer faces is that there is no one specialist to which she will automatically be referred; instead, patients tend to be passed by their general practitioner from speciality to speciality, from the gynaecologist to the psychiatrist to the physician and on to the endocrinologist.

The trouble with this is that no one specialist stands back and takes a look at the whole woman – each is interested only in his or her own speciality. It is this need for a *holistic* approach that has led to the emergence of alternative medicine for the treatment of PMS (see Chapter 7).

Mary, aged 35, came with a carefully written list of an amazing 53 symptoms! However, a look at her chart soon revealed that some of these problems were occurring every day, with no freedom from symptoms after her period. She had daily depression, facial hairs, dry skin and splitting nails, although the breast tenderness and bloatedness only occurred in the premenstruum. She complained that eight different consultants had not taken her problem seriously, and each had referred her on to another department in the hospital. Most of her symptoms were clearly not due to PMS; the last-mentioned seemingly were – either way, what the poor woman needed, but did not find, was someone who would look at her and her problems as a *whole* instead of prescribing medication for, say, the skin condition alone and passing her on to the next specialist to deal with her next problem.

This spread of symptoms over many specialities is found with all hormonal diseases, for hormones are chemical messengers and are carried round the body in the blood to affect many different types of tissue. For instance, in diabetes there may be weight loss; loss of energy; increased tendency to bacterial, fungal and viral infections as well as high blood pressure, heart and eye problems. Diabetics also tend to go to many specialists before their diabetes is diagnosed.

It is also characteristic of hormonal diseases for both psychological and bodily symptoms to occur together. For instance, excess of thyroid hormone is characterized by anxiety and restlessness in addition to loss of weight, continual heat and moist skin. Insufficient thyroid results in lethargy and depression, as well as weight gain, continual coldness and dry, coarse skin.

OTHERS SUFFER, TOO

The wide variety of the psychological symptoms that can occur with PMS means that it not only affects the woman herself, but also her partner, parents, children, friends, neighbours and workmates. Indirectly it affects all sorts of people and needs to be recognized and understood not only by the medical, nursing and caring professions, but also by the social services, police, lawyers, magistrates, teachers and youth workers, as well as by employers and managers in offices and factories.

Certainly not all PMS sufferers are criminals, but a large number of female criminals suffer from PMS. These people can be treated to become useful citizens, rather than spending their days in prison at the taxpayer's expense (see Chapter 15, for Nicola's story). At the same time, of course, it is in everyone's interests that nobody gets away with a reduced sentence on a false claim of PMS. Unfortunately, this has happened a few times in recent years, although there have also been a number of well-publicized cases in which PMS was quite rightly claimed as a defence.

HOW SEVERE IS IT?

The severity of PMS varies enormously, from at the one extreme death (by suicide or murder), epileptic fits or acute asthma requiring admission to intensive care units, right down to the mildest pimple, short-lived tiredness or occasional caustic comment. Severity of PMS is not judged by how many days the symptoms last. Sometimes, as in the case of an epileptic fit, they only last a few minutes, while others (such as tiredness) may continue for up to 14 days. Nor is the severity judged by the total number of symptoms a patient can recall. It is judged, of course, by the effect that the severest symptoms have on the sufferer's life, taken as a whole.

This wide variation in the severity of PMS symptoms from a minor inconvenience to something potentially life-threatening causes problems for professionals making observations aimed at finding better methods of diagnosis and treatment for PMS. The very severe cases need treatment which cannot be delayed while day-to-day observations are being made, so that these patients cannot be studied systematically. On the other hand, the mildest cases – amounting perhaps to nothing more than a bit of irritability – are too mild for serious study. Many studies limit their observations to those whose symptoms are severe enough to have made them ask for help from a doctor or counsellor, or which have kept them off work in the previous two months.

So that's what PMS is like – what's available to treat it?

It is unfortunately true that while some of the available treatments have been recommended for a good reason, there are also those promoted by entrepreneurs hoping for a quick turn-over and knowing that their claims are unlikely to be challenged. When you buy a remedy over the counter, the typical manufacturer counts only his profit when the cash till rings. He is not really interested in you, nor does he later request

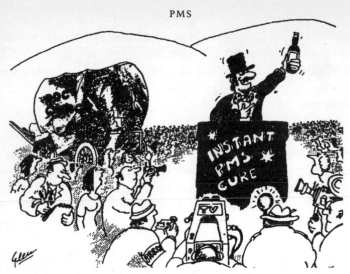

Figure 16: Dr Quack's instant PMS cures

information on whether the remedy has proved effective on all, on some or on none of your symptoms. A further problem in the UK is that vitamins, herbs and the like are classed not as drugs but as foods, and so can be sold with relative freedom.

When one realizes that PMS is a problem for at the very least one million women of menstruating age in Britain today, one appreciates why there is such a massive industry encouraging women to buy unproven remedies, whether they suffer from PMS or any other ailment. One advertisement for garlic tablets in the national press recommended them as 'working wonders' for many symptoms including premenstrual ones. An interested reader wrote asking what clinical trials there had been to substantiate the claim for PMS. The reply, on beautifully embossed paper, stated that *once* they had received a letter from a woman who said that she had benefited from the tablets. One unknown woman at some unknown time, somewhere or other, was the basis for their claims – so be warned!

PMS Help, a national charity (see Chapter 15), is constantly getting samples of such quack nostrums from manufacturers or, more commonly, public relations organizations, with a request to promote them in the charity's magazine, *PMS Helplink*. The charity routinely writes back saying that they know of no evidence for the efficacy of the product – or, often, that they know of studies showing that it doesn't work. The senders are always asked to provide the evidence, failing which the charity will advise its members not to bother with this (usually very expensive) 'cure'. As yet, no producer has ever written back. Not one.

If anyone feels at this point that I am being just a little bit paranoid about these commercial interests, she should consider the fact that after all the well-publicized tragedies, Thalidomide is still being produced today and sold in countries where the laws on medicines are not as strict as they are here in Britain. Many producers are still making – and selling – large amounts of vitamin B_6, although a number of reputable studies both here and abroad have clearly shown that even quite small excesses of this vitamin can be dangerous (see Chapter 7). What is worse, I know that in Germany the results of at least one reputable study on B_6 were suppressed after threats of legal action by a big company. A bit over the top? It happened.

Chapter 4

WHAT CAUSES PMS?

Too many articles on PMS begin with the statement that the cause is unknown, and then proceed to discuss treatment or the results of clinical trials. I agree that this was true – the cause was unknown – when the words 'Premenstrual Syndrome' first appeared in medical literature in May 1953. (This was by Dr Raymond Greene and Dr Katharina Dalton, in the *British Medical Journal*.) Scientific medicine was only just beginning and finding the evidence; the diagnosis and the cause of the disease depended largely on observation, clinical examination (which it is now fashionable to regard as 'anecdotal') and primitive blood and urine examinations. Those were the days before electron microscopes, ultrasound scanning, radioimmunoassays, chromatography, genetic imaging and all the other new technologies.

Today, editors of medical journals prefer articles on treatment and results of clinical trials rather than papers discussing the possible causes of disease. This was particularly true in the study of the hormones controlling menstruation, but work went ahead very rapidly when scientists saw that it might be possible to develop an oral contraceptive using the sex hormones. The Pill has, of course, been with us for a long time now and has been responsible for a major change in sexual habits in the Western world, as well as providing women with a simple way out of the nightmare of constant childbearing. It might not be too cynical to add that many researchers were also spurred on by the obvious consideration that the Pill would be one of the biggest money-spinners of all time – which it has been. Later, research into the female sex hormones was needed in pursuit of other work such as the development of treatments for infertility, and *in vitro* fertilization. Nowadays there is a whole new speciality of 'Gynaecological Endocrinology', which is the study not only of the levels of hormones in the blood but is concerned with their activity and chemical interactions within the nucleus of cells where the genes and chromosomes are situated. Studies are continuing world-wide, not only on humans but on all animal species, to unravel the mysteries of disease and normality. The study of PMS is no exception, and there are international meetings of scientists and doctors at which the latest knowledge and research results are shared and discussed.

THE MENSTRUAL CYCLE

To discover why the symptoms of PMS occur only before menstruation and disappear after menstruation, we need to understand the purpose of menstruation and what happens to the hormones in the different stages of the menstrual cycle.

The main purpose of the cycle is to prepare for pregnancy and reproduction. About 14 days after menstruation starts there is the release of an ovum (or egg cell) from the ovary; this is called 'ovulation'. At this time the pregnancy hormone *progesterone* (also produced in the ovary) is released into the blood.

While the ovum is making its way towards the womb, in order to be fertilized by a sperm from the male, the progesterone is carried round the body in the blood and passes to the womb, where it helps to thicken the lining of the womb to make a nice comfortable spot for the fertilized ovum, or embryo, to attach itself. If pregnancy occurs the embryo grows, a placenta is formed and there is a massive increase in progesterone. However, if the ovum is not fertilized pregnancy does not follow, the progesterone production stops and the thickened lining of the womb disintegrates and is shed through the vagina as menstrual blood. In fact, menstruation is a sign that pregnancy has failed, and another attempt is made the following month. In short,

---

Menstruation is failed pregnancy.

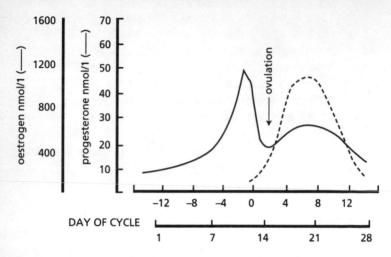

Figure 17: Levels of oestrogen and progesterone throughout the menstrual cycle

After menstruation, when the lining of the womb has been shed, a new lining appears – initially under the influence of oestrogen – and at ovulation this lining is further thickened by the introduction of progesterone. The levels of these two menstrual hormones are shown in Figure 17. You will note that oestrogen is present in varying amounts throughout the cycle, whereas progesterone is only present from ovulation to menstruation.

Figure 17 shows the levels in an average menstrual cycle of 28 days, but I have already emphasized that a normal healthy cycle can last from 21 to 36 days (page 10). Nevertheless, ovulation usually occurs not more than 14 days before menstruation, which means it does not always occur on Day 14 but may come at any time between Day 10 and Day 22, depending on the length of the individual woman's normal cycle.

The Menstrual Controlling Centre

The organization of reproduction in women is carried out at the *menstrual controlling centre* in the hypothalamus at the base of the brain (Figure 6, page 17). This is a part of the brain which also contains the controlling centres for day/night rhythm, weight control and mood control. Here a hormone called *gonadotrophin releasing hormone* (or GnRH) passes from the menstrual controlling centre to the nearby *pituitary gland*, situated just below the brain.

The pituitary gland secretes many different hormones with varying functions, controlling growth and the activities of the adrenal glands, pancreas and kidneys, but most important for us it also secretes hormones which stimulate the ovaries. There are two pituitary-ovarian stimulating hormones. One is *follicle stimulating hormone* (FSH), which stimulates an immature egg cell in an ovary to mature and also stimulates the ovary to produce *oestrogen*. The oestrogen acts on the womb to replace the lining, which was shed at the previous menstruation.

About 14 days after menstruation started there is a sudden release of another pituitary/ovarian hormone, *luteinizing hormone* (LH), which stimulates the now mature egg cell, or ovum, to be released at ovulation, and also to produce the pregnancy hormone *progesterone*, which thickens up the lining of the womb (Figure 17). This is the reason for calling the first half of the cycle the 'follicular phase', when FSH is the predominant hormone, and the second half of the cycle the 'luteinizing phase', when LH is the predominant hormone. At each stage there is a feedback mechanism, so that all the organs involved in reproduction are aware of what is going on in other parts of the chain of events (Figure 18).

If the ovum is fertilized by sperm from the male and conception occurs, a message passes to the menstrual controlling centre and almost immediately the output of hormones is changed. There is an immediate increase in the levels of progesterone and oestrogen, and there is also the secretion of new hormones, the *chorionic gonadotrophin hormones*. These lead to the formation of a new hormone-producing factory, the *placenta*, which (among other things) produces massive quantities of progesterone, some 40 or 50 times the amount normally produced during the peak level of the menstrual cycle.

This high level of progesterone continues throughout the nine months of pregnancy. At birth, after the baby is born, the placenta also comes away. This causes a dramatic drop in the progesterone level, and within 24 hours it is down to the blood level normally found in the menstrual cycle (see Figure 11, page 24).

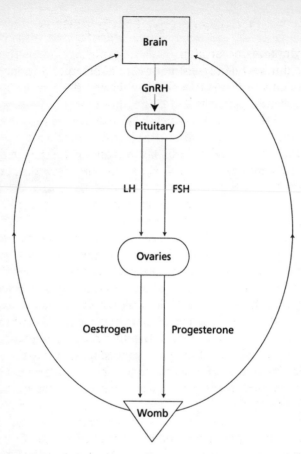

Figure 18: Hormonal pathway from the brain to the womb

During pregnancy another hormone, *prolactin*, is produced, whose function is to prepare the breasts for lactation, or milk production. Prolactin continues to be secreted at a high level as long as breastfeeding continues – it is stimulated by the baby's sucking. While the prolactin level is raised during breastfeeding, menstruation does not usually occur. Menstruation and ovulation usually restart after breastfeeding has finished and the prolactin level drops. For this reason the old belief that breastfeeding prevents pregnancy is essentially true, though it is not wise to rely on it as a means of contraception!

Timing of PMS Symptoms

PMS symptoms occur after ovulation and until menstruation – just the times when progesterone should be present in the blood. PMS goes away during pregnancy when there is a very high level of progesterone.

Following pregnancy, postnatal depression may occur in some 10 per cent of new mothers – this is the time when there is the sudden abrupt drop in the blood progesterone level. PMS may increase in severity or may occur for the first time after a pregnancy, after there has been a massive rise and sudden drop in the progesterone level. Considering these facts about the timing of PMS symptoms, it is not surprising that early researchers suspected that progesterone was involved in causing PMS. In the 1950s we did not have a quick and easy way to measure the blood progesterone level; instead the breakdown product of progesterone (called *pregnanediol*) was measured in the urine. It was known that some of the pregnanediol was excreted in the faeces as well as in the urine, so the test was not very reliable. Now we have tests called radioimmunoassays, so sensitive and reliable estimations of blood progesterone levels are possible. These tests show that there are no differences in the levels of progesterone in normal women and those with PMS. Furthermore there are no differences in the levels of any of the other hormones related to menstruation, such as oestrogen, FSH, LH, aldactide or prolactin between normal and PMS women.

There was one exception, noted by Dr Maureen Dalton in the 1980s, which was the low level of *Sex Hormone Binding Globulin* (SHBG) in 50 women with severe PMS, compared with 50 normal women (Figure 19). She also noted that there was a dose-dependent rise in the SHBG level when progesterone was given (Figure 20), but in those days we could not understand where all this fitted in the search for the cause of PMS. Now we know that in spite of its name, the low SHBG level is more an indication that there is too much insulin in the blood (*hyperinsulinaemia*). Therefore SHBG is low in those women who cannot go long intervals without food because their blood sugar drops. This fact is vitally important, and I will discuss it further in Chapter 6.

47

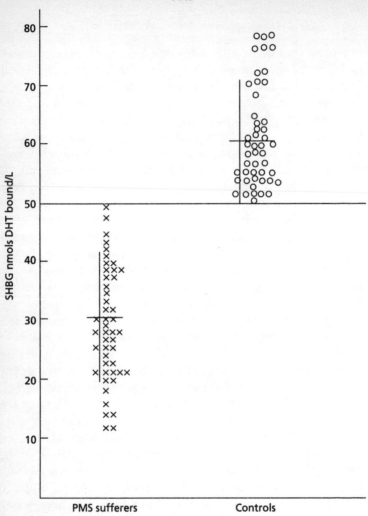

Figure 19: SHBG binding capacity in 50 patients with severe PMS and 50 controls

This test is only accurate under certain rigorous conditions. It must be performed on women who have had no medication for seven days (including vitamins, laxatives and analgesics) and no hormonal preparations for one month (including the Pill). The woman must not be unduly fat or excessively hairy and she must be free from any disease of the kidneys, liver or thyroid. So,

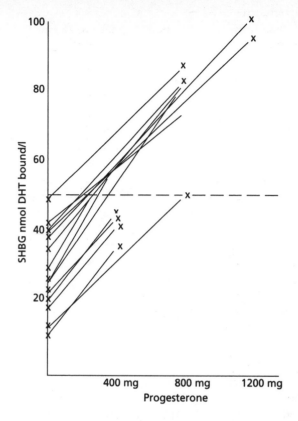

Figure 20: Rise in SHBG levels in PMS patients given progesterone therapy

while the test is not generally very useful for the diagnosis of PMS, the implications must be considered in the search for the cause of PMS.

HORMONE RECEPTORS

Scientists working with the electron microscope have revolutionized medicine, as they have been able to work out the actions which occur inside the nuclei of cells. In the 1940s we were taught as students that all cells have a nucleus, seen as a dark spot when the cells are stained and observed under a

49

microscope, but we never had any idea of the importance of this nucleus. Today we have a new branch of science, nuclear medicine, and large numbers of molecular biologists are trying to interpret their evidence of what goes on within the cell nucleus. In this book I will limit the discussion to their findings in relation to hormones, particularly progesterone.

The action of a hormone, including progesterone, takes place when a molecule of the hormone reaches the nucleus of a cell. Not all the cells in the body are designed to react to all the hormones, but for every hormone there are certain 'target' cells which will take in molecules of the hormone and then do whatever that particular hormone 'tells' them to do. (Remember, hormones are 'chemical messengers', sent out by one particular part of the body to signal to the target cells in other places to take a certain action.) In the case of progesterone, there are a lot of target cells in certain parts of the brain; also in the nose, throat and lungs; genital organs and breasts – precisely the areas in which PMS symptoms are most commonly found!

Progesterone molecules can pass through the walls of a target cell into the *cytoplasm* (the substance inside the cell), but on their own cannot get from there to the nucleus of the cell. Molecules are taken there by special compounds called 'progesterone receptors' which transport them through the substance inside the cell and into the nucleus, where the hormone does its work and is broken down (Figure 21). It is not enough just to have a high level of the hormone in the blood – to do its job it must get to the target cells, latch on ('bind') to a receptor and be carried inside the cell and on to the nucleus. The chemical formula of progesterone receptors has been discovered and molecular biologists have been able to recognize some unique characteristics in these receptors. We now have a good deal of evidence for believing that these receptors are involved with PMS.

Some very interesting work has been done by a scientist called Bruce Nock and his colleagues in New York, who have shown that progesterone receptors do not transport molecules of progesterone into the nucleus of cells if adrenalin is present, as for example when there has been a drop in the level of glucose (sugar) in the blood. This explains why dietary changes (as discussed in Chapter 6) are of importance. Another finding is that

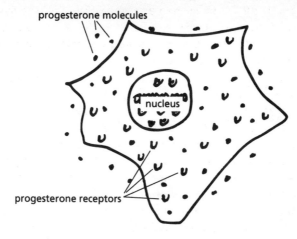

Figure 21: Cell with progesterone receptors

the progesterone receptors will not transfer the synthetic (man-made) progestogens into the nucleus of cells. This explains the failure of progestogens in the treatment of PMS (Chapter 10). Also, Blaustein and his team working in Amherst, Massachusetts have shown that while the first dose of progesterone can be very small and still act on the nucleus, later doses need to be some 40 times higher to stimulate action. In short, after the initial dose of progesterone, the subsequent chemical reaction in the nucleus becomes much less sensitive (hyposensitive) and needs a very high dose to stimulate it (see Table 2 below). This explains why high doses of progesterone are required in treating PMS and why so many double-blind controlled trials of progesterone have failed (Chapter 14).

Table 2: Unique Characteristics of Progesterone Receptors

- They do not transport progesterone if blood sugar is low.
- They do not transport synthetic progestogens.
- High doses of progesterone are required after the first dose.

The ongoing work into progesterone receptors is fascinating. In humans, progesterone receptors are already present in the fetus before birth, and their activity continues throughout life in both

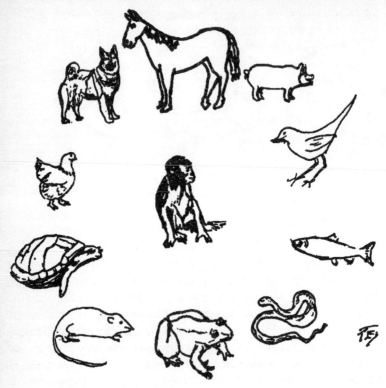

Figure 22: Animals requiring progesterone receptors

sexes. Progesterone receptors are found in all vertebrates: that is, animals with a backbone, including fish, birds, lizards and snakes as well as the well-known laboratory animals such as the guinea pig and the mouse (Figure 22). We now know that progesterone is some 500 million years old on the evolutionary scale, which means that it existed in animals over 250 million years *before* the dinosaurs ruled the Earth!

We tend to think of progesterone only as a menstrual and pregnancy hormone, essential to reproduction; we know that the blood progesterone level rises some 40 or 50 times higher during pregnancy compared with the peak level in the luteal ('PMS') phase of the menstrual cycle (see Figure 11, page 24), but we tend to forget or neglect the other important functions which it has in men as well as women. Progesterone does not play a part in reproduction of the species in the lower animals, in whom the job of progesterone is to keep the blood sugar level steady and to build up the bones as well as play a part in brain chemistry and the development of intelligence. In the adrenal glands progesterone is converted into oestrogens, testosterone and the stress hormones (e.g. cortisone).

Functions of progesterone

- Blood sugar regulation
- Brain chemistry
- Building bones
- Development of intelligence
- Reproduction
- Conversion to oestrogens, testosterones and cortisones
- Temperature control

We have already seen that, in humans, progesterone receptors are widespread and are found in the cells of all the tissues in which symptoms of PMS occur. The largest concentration of progesterone receptors is in the limbic area of the midbrain, which is the area animal physiologists call the area of rage and violence because of the rapid rage response if this particular part of the brain is stimulated.

This rage response is well known in PMS, with sudden aggression, uncontrolled irritability and mood swings, which are among the commonest of all PMS symptoms. Another common PMS symptom is headaches, and progesterone receptors are present in the meninges, or lining covering the brain, which is involved in headaches. Progesterone receptors are found in the respiratory centre in the brain and in the nose and the nasopharyngeal passages as well as the lungs. This accounts for cyclical sore throats, rhinitis, sinusitis, pharyngitis, laryngitis and asthma. They are also found in the optic pathway in the brain, which accounts for the many eye symptoms often associated with PMS. The skin, bones and bladder, as well as the womb, ovaries and Fallopian tubes all have progesterone receptors which can cause problems in the premenstruum (Figure 23).

Nowadays the molecular biologists are beginning to appreciate the part that progesterone plays in brain chemistry, and have

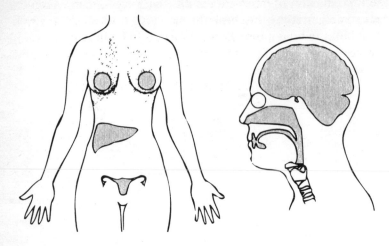

Figure 23: Sites of progesterone receptors

shown that progesterone acts as a 'monoamine oxidase inhibitor', or MAOI (a sort of natural antidepressant), and is also involved in the metabolism of dopamine and serotonin, both chemicals known to play a part in depression. (See 'antidepressants', Chapter 8; more information is to be found in 'The Aetiology of PMS is with the Progesterone Receptors' [*Medical Hypothesis*, Vol 31 Dr K. Dalton, May 1989].)

More recently, one particular biological compound called a stress protein – this one is named 'hsp 90' – has been found inside cells. It seems that its function is to regulate the number of progesterone receptors within the cells. Time will tell exactly where this particular piece of the jigsaw fits into the overall picture of progesterone's many functions, and it is highly likely that a lot more pieces will soon be discovered.

PMS AND PND

I have already mentioned the close relationship between postnatal depression (PND) and PMS (see Chapter 2). Both disorders occur when the level of progesterone in the blood drops (Figure 11, page 24). When PMS occurs after postnatal depression, the same symptoms experienced in the PND tend to return in the premenstruum as PMS: symptoms such as depression, anxiety, insomnia or paranoia. Both PND and PMS can be cured by prophylactic progesterone therapy – giving progesterone early, in time to stop them before they happen.

Maternal Behaviour in Rodents

If you take newborn rats and mice away from their mother and place them a few inches away in the cage, the mother will immediately go to her babies and care for them – she will feed, clean and provide warmth and protection for her pups. This maternal behaviour does not occur naturally in what biologists call 'naïve virgin rodents', who show no interest in newborn pups placed near them. But if such virgin rodents are given a course of oestrogen and progesterone and these hormones are then stopped, they develop maternal behaviour and start to look after the newborn pups. Thus – in rodents – maternal behaviour is under hormonal control. Maternal behaviour can also be induced in sheep and monkeys by a course of oestrogen and progesterone.

Progesterone Antibodies

Wang, Heap and Taussig in San Diego, California have learned how to immunize rats and mice so that they develop antibodies to progesterone, and if a mother has progesterone antibodies she will not look after newborn pups and may even attack them. What is more, this rejection and cannibalism will even continue after a second, normal pregnancy – once the mother has progesterone antibodies, they are there to stay.

All this is very similar to the behaviour of human mothers with PND, who often reject their babies or, in extreme cases, harm them or even kill them, and there is a high chance that postnatal depression will recur in women who have suffered from it once. It is also not unlike some of the feelings commonly experienced in PMS, which can also lead a woman to hurt her children or other loved ones. We need to know more about these progesterone antibodies; in particular, whether they occur in humans as well and, if so, what causes them and how to eliminate them.

In this short chapter I can do no more than glance at just the more important work which has been done on hormones in recent years. There are over 25,000 scientific journals published in the world. Nobody can possibly read more than a tiny fraction of this output but, like many workers in medicine and science, I subscribe to an agency which sends me all the relevant scientific papers: I receive details of over a 100 such papers every month, each one giving the results of an experiment or a clinical trial into PMS or with progesterone, on animals or humans. Some of these papers are of more interest than others, of course, but I find so many which fill in yet another small space in the jigsaw. There are areas yet untouched, we don't yet pretend to know everything about PMS – but don't worry! We do already know a lot about its causes, and nowadays we certainly do have very effective ways of treating it. These will now form the subjects of the following chapters.

PART II

Treatment Methods

Chapter 5

SELF-HELP

Some people feel that if we suggest self-help methods for PMS we are harming sufferers by implying that PMS is a minor psychological disorder which can be corrected by greater self-control, and that it is just another sign of a weak personality. This is certainly not true, as we have already seen. On the other hand, many sufferers will already have discovered for themselves that there are numerous small ways of easing or overcoming the premenstrual problems and preventing them coming to the surface and being noticed by others.

DIET

Eating the right diet is by far the most important thing you can do to help yourself beat PMS – so important that I have given it a whole chapter to itself (Chapter 6).

COPING SKILLS

It is well worth while developing your coping skills, regardless of whatever other treatment(s) you choose. Having charted your good and bad days on the menstrual chart, you will already know what your most vulnerable times are. Look again at your chart, but this time work out if the bad days often occur on a particular day of the week. You may find that weekends are usually worse, possibly because on those days you sleep longer and your blood sugar level is low by the time you get up. OK – the answer is simple: make sure you have something extra to eat immediately before you go to bed, or even put a small snack such as a biscuit by your bed to nibble when you wake up. If you haven't the energy or inclination to chew during the night (this sounds comic unless you've tried it!) how about something like custard, blancmange or rice pudding?

Maybe you are being too energetic at the weekend, trying to do too many chores to make up for having been away from home all the week. In that case, decide not to be so hard on yourself; have some extra rest at weekends. Maybe you could get some of those jobs done during the week. (Yes, I do know what I'm saying!) Twist the family's arm – maybe they'll help a bit more if they know you won't be 'PMSy' at the weekend. (What's that I hear you say? OK, so pigs don't fly all that often, but you could at least try to persuade your ever-loving partner who will benefit, too.)

If you find that a particular day of the week presents the worst problems, then again, think out the possible reasons why that might be. Do you go to bed late the previous night because you have meetings or keep-fit classes? Many mums have to drive the children back from their various activities. Or it might be the night you go to the supermarket for the weekly shopping? Is it the day the boss comes in early and stresses you, or maybe keeps you extra late? Girls, is there a particularly foul teacher who sets you a load of work on one particular day? The possible reasons are endless and very personal; our individual lives are all so different and we all interact with different people, so it becomes a personal exercise. But once you have found the reason for your bad days, think how you can avoid or ease the situation. If necessary, discuss it with your partner, parents and friends.

AVOIDANCE TACTICS

Avoidance tactics are aimed at ensuring that difficult or problem occasions do not occur in that 'bad time' before your period. For instance, consult your menstrual chart and avoid the pre-menstruum (days just before menstruation) when making an appointment with the dentist or seeing your bank manager. (Not that there's such a thing as a *good* time to see these people, but there certainly is such a thing as a *bad* time!) Try, if you possibly can, not to go for an interview, take your driving test, entertain your or your partner's boss or promise to have your project ready to hand in during the premenstruum.

Of course, it isn't nearly as easy as that in real life. Many of these things have got to happen when they happen, they can't just be put off. In that case, then, you have just got to do your best to organize the rest of your day so as tc even out the stress. Do you have an interview? Have a nice relaxing bath the night before and turn in early – blow the ironing. Is the boss coming to dinner? Get a friend or relative to help you do the shopping and cooking.

Homework? Well, even teachers can be reasonable if you talk nicely to them. You don't have to mention your PMS: make an excuse, tell the teacher you have to go and see your granny on that night and could you please have a bit more time? If not, try shifting another homework where the teacher is willing to help. In the same way, look at your menstrual chart before making important decisions like moving house, booking a holiday, changing the children's schools or altering your work schedule. Shopping for clothes, particularly shoes (as feet swell premenstrually), should definitely be organized after your period – and these are the sort of things which often can be rearranged. If you have a few days' holiday in hand, use them when you're feeling 'off'. Spoil yourself and have a really lazy time during those awkward premenstrual days – and there's no need to feel guilty! It's really just like taking medicine, and remember – if your PMS is better, the whole family is going to benefit.

When we examine the records of women who have ended up on a criminal charge due to uncontrolled PMS behaviour, we find that additional factors which increase the severity of their mood swings are tiredness, hunger, stress, alcohol and smoking, so your coping skills should include ways in which these factors can be avoided. Not that we're suggesting that you, personally, are going to end up on a criminal charge, but the underlying reasons for your PMS are likely to be the same; they are the same things which make *your* problems worse, too. (Avoidance of hunger is dealt with in Chapter 6.)

Remember, stress is not the direct cause of PMS, but it does make it worse and you are least able to cope at that time. Stress and PMS naturally aggravate each other. However busy you are, however bleak life may seem, there is almost always scope for you to do some reorganization and stress avoidance. What is very important is that you should think these things out and make your plans during your *good* days. Don't try to follow the advice given in this chapter when you are overstressed and suffering from PMS. That's asking for trouble.

AVOID NIGHT WORK

Sufferers from PMS should avoid night work; this includes evening work which entails going to bed later than your normal bedtime, as well as overnight duties – even if they do permit a snooze when things are quiet. The controlling centre for the day/night rhythm is situated in the hypothalamus, at the base of the brain adjacent to the menstrual controlling centre, so any disturbance to the day/night rhythm centre upsets the menstrual hormones. The effect is very like jet lag, when your biological clock is also disturbed. In these days of dreadfully high unemployment it is tempting to accept night work to help out the family income, but beware. It sounds so easy: your partner can cope with the children. All too often you forget that you're moonlighting, having coped with the housework, shopping, cooking and kids all day before starting your night job. It's particularly important if you're doing responsible work: driving, nursing or supervising – and don't make the excuse that you're allowed to snooze on the job. The odd snooze is not the same as proper sleep, and anyway, you never know when you will need all your wits about you.

MAKE SURE YOU GET
ENOUGH REST

The average PMS sufferer needs her full eight hours' rest in bed each night. Don't be tempted to follow the bedtimes of others in your household. When one is lying resting in bed, whether awake or fast asleep, the body works differently; in particular, the job of the kidneys is made easier. If you really can't get to sleep, don't start walking about or doing odd jobs. It's the rest in bed lying horizontally which gives you the benefit, so don't start worrying that if you're not asleep, you'll be tired the next day. It doesn't matter whether you're conscious or unconscious; it's the lack of rest which results in irritability and tiredness, not the lack of sleep. Try thinking happy thoughts, decide what you'll do when you win the pools, plan your dream holiday or wardrobe, relive some of the good events which have happened in your life. Happy thoughts only – if unpleasant ones encroach, try consciously to put them in the background and return to happy thoughts. If necessary, while dozing, have some quiet music, or you may like to listen to a relaxation tape. Insufficient rest in bed each night will make PMS worse each month.

PRACTICAL PLANNING

Use the good days after menstruation to plan ahead and avoid or ease any problems which might occur during your next premenstruum. Keep some special toys, books or puzzles hidden away so that you can keep the children out of your hair when you need peace and quiet. Hide some emergency quick meals in the freezer for use when you just can't face the extra task of cooking. At work save up simple jobs that don't need much thought, like tidying, and busy yourself with these so that no one notices it's one of your dull days when you couldn't possibly compose a sensible letter. Teachers can also prepare their lessons in advance, selecting for the premenstruum the ones that require least effort and only simple marking. Journalists will need to keep deadlines in mind, doing the simple research and interviewing in advance and, if they find the final writing up the most difficult part, ensure this is completed in their alert postmenstrual days.

EXERCISE

There is the world of difference between everyday physical exertion and beneficial exercise. When I ask women about exercise, most of them reply to the effect that 'I'm always on the go' or 'I never sit down all day.' Both of which are probably quite true, but from a doctor's point of view there is a vast difference between the 'perpetual motion' of a housewife and wholesome exercise. To be beneficial, exercise must be sufficiently prolonged to increase the pulse rate for some minutes after exercise has stopped. So, the daily chores of walking from kitchen to lounge, from bedroom to front door, from phone to dishwasher, up and down stairs, or doing the supermarket shopping do not fall into this category. What I mean by beneficial exercise would be something like 20 minutes' rhythmic activity such as working on a cycling or rowing machine, a brisk walk, a jog round the block or a hard swim. If you like, make it a competitive and/or social activity such as a game of squash, badminton, tennis or golf. Some of these suggestions are more enjoyable than others, and it's always more fun if you can exercise with others in an exercise class or at the leisure club.

Exercising is invigorating, increasing the circulation of blood and oxygen consumption. This all helps to release tension, and any premenstrual aggression is dissipated in your effort to beat the clock, your personal best or your opponent in the game – which is much better than banging pots or slamming doors! Incidentally, some studies have suggested that anaerobic exercises are better than other kinds of exercises for relieving PMS. If your only opportunity to have any exercise is the cycling machine, then put it in front of the TV and make a point of watching your favourite soap daily while pedalling away. If your children are the right age you can have a daily skipping session with them.

SELF-HELP GROUPS

These are many and various, covering the range from excellent to unmentionable, so it's very much a question of luck as to which one happens to be in your locality. It's good to be able to meet others similarly afflicted and to know that there are those who suffer worse than you. The success of a group depends largely on the leader, on her knowledge and ability to point others in the right direction to find the much-wanted relief of symptoms. Unfortunately, the leaders are very rarely qualified in medicine and so cannot understand your previous medical history and are not able to examine you or to prescribe medications. A good leader will listen to each member's story sympathetically, will show her how to chart and be able to distinguish PMS from the many other medical diagnoses (Chapter 1): she should be able to suggest self-help methods, teach the dietary regime (Chapter 6) and if necessary, know when and where she should send you to get help from the proper authority.

Each meeting should begin by reminding all present that personal disclosures and discussions will be strictly confidential. There tend to be very noticeable differences between groups: some include partners, always or sometimes, and others have their menfolk meeting separately in another room or on another day. Some take no account of the men and children at all – I feel it's essential that they do, though there can be more than one valid way of doing so. Some groups have regular meetings with definite programmes, weekly or monthly, so members gradually become more able to help themselves and others. Other groups are just 'talking shops' over a cup of tea with the blind leading the blind. These latter groups are vulnerable to unscrupulous entrepreneurs, who will try to sell unproven pills and potions, offering members discounts (which amount, therefore, to bribes).

The success of each group depends not only on the leader but on individual members, who should each be able to make her own contribution. Some individuals are too loudmouthed, too dominant, paranoid or neurotic to fit easily into a group, so that the group fails as one by one the members leave. It only needs one person to disrupt the entire group, even a well-established one. In at least one group I know of, a way has been found of overcoming this problem: they limit the number of meetings any one individual can attend.

STOP THE CONTRACEPTIVE PILL

All types of the contraceptive pill, whether the new low-dose oestrogen plus progestogen pill or the progestogen-only pill (sometimes known as the 'mini-pill'), contain an artificial drug known as a 'progestogen'. This progestogen has the effect of lowering the level of progesterone in the blood, and so increases PMS symptoms. However, if you are suffering from spasmodic dysmenorrhoea (see page 21), or have heavy periods, the Pill is likely to help with these symptoms. PMS sufferers will find more information on contraception in Chapter 13.

STOP SMOKING

By now all smokers will be well aware of the main reason for giving up smoking: it damages the lung tissue. However, for PMS sufferers there is another reason, which is that research workers have shown that smoking lowers the blood progesterone level. They did find that smoking does not cause such a drastic lowering of the progesterone blood level as taking the progestogens found in the contraceptive pill, but the effect is still bad enough to make a difference. If you are addicted to smoking, then that is yet another reason to take the vital step – try to stop. Maybe you could try the new nicotine patches, although there are now some indications that these may also cause other kinds of problem. If you are not a smoker, then there is another good reason for not starting! Incidentally, if you have PMS you must begin any attempt to give up smoking at the beginning of your 'good' days; to stop smoking premenstrually is to invite failure.

CUT DOWN ON ALCOHOL

You do not have to be a heavy drinker to make your PMS worse – a fairly small amount will do the trick. Scientists as far apart as Switzerland and Japan have shown that when alcohol is taken it interferes with the normal action of progesterone in brain chemistry, or more specifically, it lessens the ability of progesterone to break down monoamine oxidase. Remember, if you are suffering from clinical depression, one drug you are likely to be given is a *monoamine oxidase inhibitor*, or MAOI. This means that PMS sufferers who already have problems with low progesterone suffer worse symptoms when taking alcohol. They will also find that they are not able to take nearly as much alcohol as they once could without becoming intoxicated. Many PMS sufferers will confirm this from personal experience and already try to avoid alcohol altogether in the premenstruum, or at least restrict it to minimal amounts. If in doubt, look again at your menstrual chart and see if there is any increase in symptoms on those days when you have drunk alcohol.

COLOUR THERAPY

Colour therapy has been described by Dr de Vries (once a pharmacist and now in alternative medicine) as 'a marvellous therapy, which has proved of great benefit'. I must confess that I have never been fortunate enough to hear of even one success with it, nor is there any medical evidence that the colour of one's clothes influences the endocrine glands and their secretion of hormones. (A nice new dress might cheer you up, but this is not what the therapy's proponents mean.)

Seven days before a period is due, it is suggested that you should wear 'cyanogen blue' to stimulate the pituitary gland. Six days before, wear violet to buck up the pineal gland. Five days before, wear green to stimulate the thyroid, and four days before, choose yellow to wake up the thymus gland. Then for one day wear orange to act on the pancreas, and the next day orange-red to activate the adrenal glands, and finally wear red on the last premenstrual day to help the ovaries. Then the day after the period, turn up in something greeny-blue and, it is promised, 'you will feel great'.

I make no such promise; in my view it just has to be a leg-pull. Just imagine the media reaction in the Commons if Lady Thatcher had turned up in a bright red dress before her resignation! Still, you can try it if you like; it certainly won't do you any harm.

Finally: some of the suggestions in this chapter may be hard to put into practice (like a lot of the advice in this book), but with PMS you often have some hard choices to make. I'm afraid I do sometimes have to overrule people's objections by saying (as nicely as possible!) 'Well, we've told you what's needed, and in the end, I'm afraid that you're going to have to choose between . . . and being well again.' PMS is an illness. It can be very serious and it seldom gets better on its own: it generally gets worse, at least until the menopause. It's not like appendicitis, which can be fixed once and for all by a fairly straightforward operation, after which you never need give it another thought: PMS is going to be with you for a long time. You can beat it, but only by keeping on with whatever you find to be your personal solution.

Chapter 6

DIET AND PMS

The aim of this chapter is to give specific dietary advice to sufferers of PMS, not general dietary advice for good health. Even if PMS sufferers are eating a good, healthy, varied and nutritious diet containing sufficient protein, high-fibre carbohydrates, fresh fruit and vegetables, it may still be unsuitable and cause or aggravate their PMS.

The part played by progesterone receptors in the cause of PMS is discussed in Chapter 4 (and fully explained in an article in the May 1990 issue of *Medical Hypothesis*.) Among the unique characteristics of progesterone receptors is the fact that they can't transport molecules of progesterone into the nucleus of the target cells if there is no sugar in those cells (see Table 2, page 51). Since then, research has shown that after a large meal there is a temporary drop in the level of progesterone, due to an increased metabolic clearance rate of that hormone. In other words, after a heavy meal the progesterone is broken down and got rid of much more quickly. Thus, eating a heavy meal is likely to make your PMS symptoms worse for a while (Figure 24).

It is also known that if you go for a long time without food, the blood sugar level drops. To correct this low blood sugar the body releases adrenalin. What then happens is that the adrenalin makes your cells release their stored sugar into the blood, so as to raise the low blood sugar level. All cells contain sugar, and when the sugar drains out it is replaced by water. This swells up the cells, causing the sensations of bloatedness and, later, weight gain. Furthermore, adrenalin is the hormone of the 'fight, fright and flight' response – it winds you up. This is what causes the tension, depression, anxiety and irritability experienced by so many PMS sufferers.

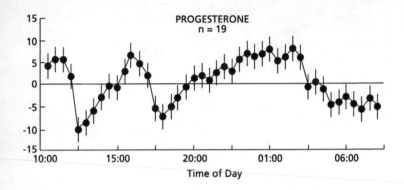

Figure 24: Progesterone levels after large meals

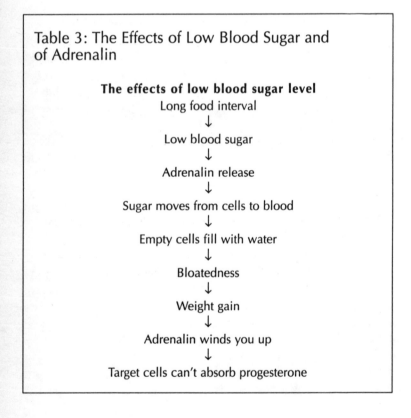

Table 3: The Effects of Low Blood Sugar and of Adrenalin

The effects of low blood sugar level

Long food interval
↓
Low blood sugar
↓
Adrenalin release
↓
Sugar moves from cells to blood
↓
Empty cells fill with water
↓
Bloatedness
↓
Weight gain
↓
Adrenalin winds you up
↓
Target cells can't absorb progesterone

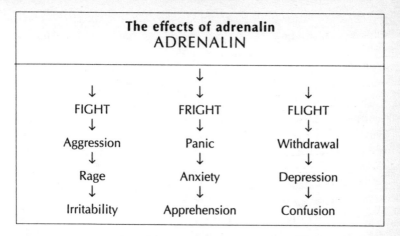

The effects of adrenalin ADRENALIN		
↓	↓	↓
FIGHT	FRIGHT	FLIGHT
↓	↓	↓
Aggression	Panic	Withdrawal
↓	↓	↓
Rage	Anxiety	Depression
↓	↓	↓
Irritability	Apprehension	Confusion

THE THREE-HOURLY STARCH DIET

To overcome the problem of low blood sugar, it is important for PMS sufferers to keep their blood sugar level steady throughout the day. The essential rule is to divide the normal day's diet into about six snacks, ensuring that each snack contains some starch, and always to eat within one hour of waking and one hour of going to bed. As well as the starch, the diet should contain a good and varied selection of foods to supply protein, vitamins and minerals.

The Three-hourly Starch Diet

- Eat small starchy snacks every three hours throughout the day.
- Always eat within one hour of waking up.
- Always eat a snack one hour or less before you go to bed.
- Continue with a healthy, varied and nutritious diet.

Starchy foods are:

- Flour
- Potatoes
- Oats
- Rice
- Maize
- Rye

It does not matter what other foods are eaten at the same snack. Cheese can still be eaten with the crackers; eggs, fish and salad in the sandwiches; meat and vegetables with a potato, as well as fruit, fresh vegetables and yoghurt. But *please note:* it is the *starch* that matters; it is a type of carbohydrate that raises the blood sugar level for about three hours, before it drops.

Sugar is also a carbohydrate, but when you eat sugar or chocolate on its own there is a rapid rise in blood sugar level followed by a 'rebound' fall, causing yet more trouble. As for the fashionable high-fibre carbohydrates – these may keep the blood sugar level steady once it is high enough, but they do not necessarily raise it sufficiently if it is low.

This is the only dietary rule which is important to sufferers of PMS, regardless of whether their symptoms are mild, moderate or severe, or whether they suffer psychologically, physically or both. It is also essential for women to follow this three-hourly starch diet when taking progesterone, otherwise the progesterone cannot do its job. Furthermore, the three-hourly diet needs to be continued *throughout the entire cycle*, day after day, and month after month until it becomes such a habit you don't even know you're doing it.

This three-hourly starch habit is quite easy for those who already eat a good, normal diet. Write down what you ate yesterday or what you usually eat. Underline all the starch foods, then divide these starch foods into six or seven snacks, making sure that you have one within an hour of getting up in the morning and one an hour or less before going to bed.

When it comes to foods, we all have our different likes and dislikes, we need different amounts and have different mealtimes, so each individual woman needs to plan the diet to suit her personally. Try to have roughly the same amount of starch at each snack. In your main meal, try to limit the starch to just one medium-sized potato or equivalent, so that you have more starch during the rest of the day. It is a 'nibbling' or 'grazing' diet, different from the typical diet which is generally a 'gorging' diet with only one or two big meals each day.

Typically this means halving the toast at breakfast and having the remaining half at elevenses, or substituting a biscuit or crispbread. Your lunchtime sandwich can be halved (you can still have the usual apple or yoghurt) and then you have the other half of the sandwich in the mid-afternoon. At supper, save the fruit tart to have at bedtime, or substitute some toast, biscuits or crispbreads. If you are eating the same amount of food, divided into snacks, you won't put on extra weight. In fact, if it cures the premenstrual cravings for sweet things, or 'bingeing' which affects so many sufferers, those people who need to lose weight will be surprised how easy it is to shed the extra pounds. Also, remember that the starch foods do not have the high calories contained in fats and sugars. For example, a crispbread contains about 25 calories, so six crispbreads a day only add up to 150 calories.

A word of warning: it is starch that matters, not carbohydrate or even high-fibre carbohydrate. Did you know that one biscuit contains as much starch as 12 bananas or 12 apples? So don't try substituting fruit for starch. I am not saying that high-fibre foods are not helpful in other ways, just that fibre won't do instead of starch when it comes to the ideal diet for PMS.

Following this diet involves no extra cost and little or no change in the foods you normally eat, but it does need self-discipline. The hardest time is at the beginning; once it becomes a habit, it is no problem. If you're not a clock-watcher, it may be a good idea to have a watch with an alarm that you can set to go off every three hours to remind you. If you are off to a meeting which might last three hours, then eat just before you go in, even if it's not yet three hours since your last snack. If the meeting continues for more than three hours, it is quite acceptable to ask to be excused so that you can nibble your snack in peace. If you can't, then you can always nip off to the toilet.

It's also important to carry a starchy snack with you in your handbag, as you never know when there will be a delay on your journey or some other unforeseen problem to catch you out. In the US many PMS self-help groups start their meetings by asking folk to open their handbags and reveal their hidden snacks!

Avoid Sugar

When you eat sugar without any starch, as in a chocolate bar or in tea or coffee, the sugar is absorbed into your bloodstream very rapidly. This makes the blood sugar level shoot up, and – unless you are so unfortunate as to be a diabetic – your body produces insulin to cope with the extra-high level. Down goes the blood sugar level again, which results in a release of adrenalin and all the problems mentioned earlier. This is called *rebound hypoglycaemia* and is a well-known effect. So it is important not to have sugar alone, although there is no harm in having some sugar with starch. The sugar causes a rapid rise in blood sugar level, but the starch, keeps the blood sugar level up.

Binges and Food Cravings

I mentioned earlier that one common feature among PMS sufferers is their tendency to binge or have food cravings during the premenstruum. Binges occur when too much sugar has been removed from the body's cells and the brain sends out urgent messages to your body to eat everything in sight so as to get some sugar back into the cells.

When you have the urge to binge, the right thing to do is to give way and binge to your heart's content to replenish the sugar in your body's cells. There's no need to feel guilty. The craving isn't there for nothing: every cell in your body needs sugar – give them some, *this time*. But promise yourself that it will never happen again. The desire to binge will only happen if you have deprived yourself of starch, either having had too long a food gap, or because over several days you've been having less starch than your body really needs. Work out what caused it and ensure that another binge never happens.

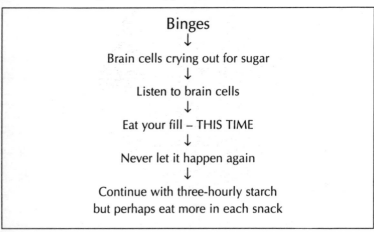

Binges
↓
Brain cells crying out for sugar
↓
Listen to brain cells
↓
Eat your fill – THIS TIME
↓
Never let it happen again
↓
Continue with three-hourly starch
but perhaps eat more in each snack

The Effectiveness of the Three-hourly Starch Diet

In 1992, findings were reported by myself and Mrs Wendy Holton in the medical journal *Stress Medicine* of a study concerning 84 women with severe PMS. The women had completed a questionnaire giving particulars of all the food they ate during seven consecutive days, and the exact times at which they ate it. I don't mean that they did this from memory – that wouldn't be very reliable; they did it for a week after they received the questionnaire, filling it out a day at a time.

They were asked to do this while waiting for an appointment to see the specialist about their PMS. That means that they were all quite severe cases, because they could only ask for an appointment if they had been referred to the specialist by their doctor. The results showed that only 51 per cent regularly had any breakfast (Figure 25).

What is worse, the average food gap was over five hours during the day and over 12 hours overnight. In fact, only one woman was eating regular three-hourly starch (Figure 26).

When they returned their questionnaires, they were advised to stick to the three-hourly starch diet for the rest of the time until they got to see the specialist. (Unfortunately, the waiting list was

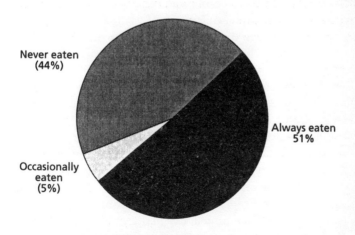

Figure 25: PMS sufferers who eat breakfast

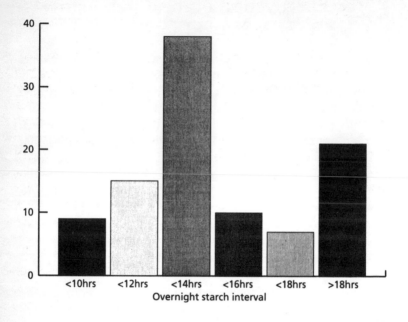

Figure 26: Overnight food gaps in women with PMS

several months.) When they arrived, the specialist asked them whether they had in fact stuck to the diet, and whether they had improved. Later on in the interview, the specialist had to sort out whether they did in fact have PMS. Although referred by a doctor, some of them did not have PMS. The ones with PMS had excellent results, better than those with menstrual distress (Figure 27).

Several patients began the interview by saying that they had only come to thank the specialist, they didn't need help any more. Some cancelled their appointments for the same reason; this unfortunately meant that they had to be taken out of the study, which brought down the percentage of the women who could be shown to have benefited! Even so, over 64 per cent got a lot of benefit and another 25 per cent noticed some improvement. That adds up to 90 per cent of PMS sufferers helped by the diet. We now know that the figures are better still if the patients with less improvement are also given progesterone, but I'll discuss that in detail in Chapter 11.

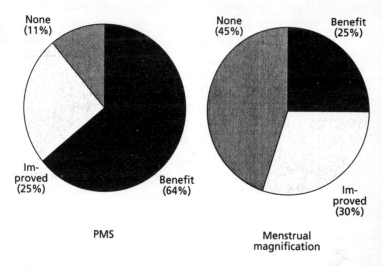

None
(11%)

None
(45%)

Benefit
(25%)

Im-
proved
(25%)

Benefit
(64%)

Im-
proved
(30%)

PMS

Menstrual
magnification

Figure 27: Effect of three-hourly starch diet on PMS and menstrual distress (magnification)

UNNECESSARY FOOD RESTRICTIONS

In the rest of this chapter we are going to have a look at some cases of 'hearsay' – things to do with food which you often hear mentioned in connection with PMS, but which in fact have little or nothing to do with it.

Avoid Tea and Coffee?

Tea, coffee and cola drinks contain caffeine, and so all of them have a stimulating effect just after you drink them. Later on, though, there is a reaction and you then feel drowsy. This can mean that some women – and men – feel an increase in tension for a while and, if you drink these beverages late in the day, they may stop you getting to sleep. Some people are more sensitive to caffeine than others when it comes to its stimulating action, while others are more affected by the restlessness and insomnia. What is worse, caffeine is also quite addictive; some people can find it very hard to cut down or give up. There are people who drink 20 or even 40 cups of coffee a day, and who therefore naturally get restless and tense. These addicts should be advised to break their addiction, just as other addicts are advised to stop alcohol, smoking, drugs or gambling.

Strictly speaking, all this has nothing to do with the treatment of PMS, for the effect of caffeine and the tendency to addiction are due to a personal sensitivity which remains the same throughout the menstrual cycle. However, those unfortunate people who are affected by caffeine and suffer tension, agitation, anxiety or insomnia would be well advised to avoid drinking too much tea, coffee or cola, and if necessary to cut them out altogether, especially late in the day. Caffeine does not affect other PMS symptoms.

It is worthwhile finding out your personal reaction to caffeine by noting the difference when you have caffeine, compared to the way you feel after a few days without it. Incidentally, it doesn't matter whether you drink your tea or coffee with or without milk, as it is the amount of caffeine that counts. Coffee has more caffeine than tea, and some brands of each contain more caffeine than others.

Avoid Yeast?

You often read that PMS sufferers should avoid foods containing yeast. Even healthy people naturally have a lot of yeasts in their intestines, where, together with bacteria, they help with normal digestion. Yeasts generally cause no problems so long as they remain in the intestines, but trouble does arise when the yeasts, particularly one type called 'candida', get into the vagina, mouth or other parts of the body, causing a condition known as 'thrush' or 'candidiasis'. Once in the vagina, the candida can be transmitted during sexual intercourse and so the male partner becomes infected. Perhaps unfairly, the male is frequently unaware of the infection and is just a symptomless carrier who passes it back to the female after she has been successfully treated. Treatment of candidiasis has changed in the last year or two: the patient and her partner now need to take just one capsule of a medicine called fluconazole (UK brand name Diflucan), and in the vast majority of cases the candidiasis disappears completely in the next few days.

Every baker knows that yeast is killed by heat, so there is no logical reason for PMS sufferers to avoid eating yeast in foods such as bread, which have been cooked and therefore have no live yeast in them. Even if there were a problem with eating yeast, it would not be restricted to women with PMS.

Avoid Salt?

Before doctors knew that the bloatedness often experienced in PMS was caused by a low blood sugar level, women were often advised to reduce their salt intake. Today we understand that bloatedness can be prevented by following the three-hourly starch diet, and cutting down on salt is not necessary – not to cure PMS, anyway.

Avoid Wheat and Other Specific Foods?

There are some individuals who are allergic or sensitive to certain foods, and they are often advised to avoid *wheat*, *dairy products*, *citrus fruits*, *chocolate*, *onions*, *strawberries* or whatever. If you really do have such an allergy, it will affect you throughout the month, although you may find that your reaction may be more severe during the premenstruum.

In short, if you do have such an allergy – and it is rarer than people often think – it is not caused by PMS, though it just might make your PMS worse. Therefore, in spite of what we are often told, there is no reason whatsoever why all PMS sufferers should be advised to avoid certain foods. After all, we don't advise everybody to avoid sugar just because people who have diabetes can't tolerate it.

There are some expensive blood tests (Mast and Rast) which will determine whether you are allergic to many common food items. Often it is an unsuspected item which shows up on the test, such as soya flour or peanuts, and then it is advisable to eliminate that specific item completely from your diet. Another blood test can measure your IgE, a special protein called an 'immunoglobulin' which has to do with allergies. This test measures how allergic you are in general. If your IgE test result is low, then it is unlikely that food allergy is your problem. If your IgE is high, then it is worthwhile trying to find out the cause of your allergy.

Alternatively, if you feel that certain food items may be the cause of your problems, you could keep a written list, called an *attack form*, of all foods you have consumed during the 24 hours immediately before an attack of symptoms such as a migraine, panic or breathlessness (Table 1, page 30). After you have collected three or more such forms you may well notice one specific food item which you ate on the day before each attack. It is then worth cutting out that item completely from your food for a month or more. If you then eat that food again and it again causes trouble, you will know that you have tracked down the cause of your problems, and the answer will be to avoid it completely in future.

Chapter 7

TREATMENT WITHOUT DRUGS

This chapter deals with treatments which do not rely on drugs and which have all at one time or another been recommended for PMS, as well as for numerous other diseases in both men and women. In other words, they are not aimed at curing PMS or even treating PMS alone, but they are supposed to cure certain general troubles, such as depression, which can be a part of PMS. Many of the treatments mentioned here are excellent for other diseases, but not necessarily for PMS, and it is to help PMS sufferers that this chapter (and this book) has been written.

Britain has an advertising code which prohibits advertising to the public treatments for a list of 'recognized diseases'. This list includes diseases such as cancer, heart and kidney failure; the sort of diseases which need medical treatment and which may be made worse if unproven remedies are tried. It was only recently that 'premenstrual syndrome' was added to this list. So, PMS is now regarded as a specific disease, but it is still legal to advertise treatment for the relief of symptoms such as dysmenorrhoea (or period pains). What is more, journalists are allowed to advocate treatments in their columns, which are not regarded as advertisements – just another loophole in the law. Just today I was looking at a daily newspaper – and a fairly 'respectable' one, at that – which contained full-page articles on real or imaginary diseases, with so-called cures. It's the same every day, and I don't mean just that one paper.

The treatments advocated in this chapter are essentially for the relief of the symptoms of PMS, aiming to help with the miseries of depression, tension, irritability and tiredness without removing the underlying cause. If you suffer most from physical problems such as premenstrual asthma, skin or eye complaints, cystitis, bingeing, breast tenderness or bloatedness, you may prefer to miss out this chapter.

Many non-drug treatments are recommended by men and those fortunate women who have never suffered from PMS. The treatments are based on the idea that the PMS symptoms are 'all in the mind', and can be helped by the woman 'pulling herself together', rather than appreciating that PMS is a hormonal disease needing hormonal treatment.

MORE THAN ONE SYMPTOM

A characteristic of hormonal diseases in general, and PMS in particular, is that the unfortunate individual has several different complaints at the same time and these complaints involve many different systems or parts of the body. This is not surprising when one appreciates that the hormones are passed into the blood and so go all over the body. Common examples include the woman with premenstrual depression, backache and bloatedness or another woman with premenstrual headaches, panic attacks and acne. The treatments examined in this chapter are designed to improve the general 'Feel-Well' score, without necessarily attempting to pinpoint the source of the problem.

Clinical trials of PMS (Chapter 14) always show a high 'placebo effect', especially in the first month of any controlled trial. That means that women volunteering to enter the trials who are only given a placebo, or 'dummy' treatment, show an initial benefit. The reason for this is not really known, although it is suspected that it is because the woman is given the same attention as the one receiving the effective treatment. It may well be the first time that anyone has ever taken any notice of the woman and her problem, or that anyone has ever been interested in her and what she has to say. In short, if someone is sympathetic and listens to her many problems, that in itself will make her feel better and increase her 'Feel-Well' score. The many treatments in this chapter which are given by 'alternative' medical practitioners may, I believe, at first be effective just because of this placebo, or 'Feel-Well' response. They may be worth considering, especially if the PMS is only of mild severity.

RELAXATION

Relaxation is the recommended answer for those who are tense and unable to unwind. It is a non-specific therapy which might be useful for those suffering only from tension in the premenstruum, as well as for men and women who are tense and anxious every day of the month. Relaxation and breathing exercises are taught at antenatal classes (among others) and are helpful for women suffering from spasmodic dysmenorrhoea (see page 21), as the same nerves are involved in opening the door of the womb at a baby's birth as are needed to expel the blood at menstruation. But women with severe spasmodic dysmenorrhoea rarely have PMS.

There are relaxation tapes and cassettes available for use at home, although many prefer to attend relaxation classes where they will meet others with similar problems and when there is a set time each week to learn the art. They will still need to practise daily at home. Alternatively there are 'Relaxation for Living' teachers who give classes at home (see the Useful Addresses section). Some schools teach relaxation as part of Physical Education, or English or Drama. It is certainly an art well worth learning by all adults – its benefits can be felt by both sexes, every day of the month – but is not directly relevant to PMS.

ASSERTIVENESS TRAINING

There are some women blighted with shyness, unable to speak up for themselves about the many injustices they sustain, wanting to hide in a corner, afraid to be seen, spoken to or even noticed. These characteristics are invariably present throughout the cycle, and very rarely are they limited to the premenstruum alone. Assertion classes are aimed at overcoming these problems; in Britain they are usually run by Community Psychiatric Nurses (CPNs). If you feel you come into this category and are likely to benefit from assertiveness training, you will need to ask your general practitioner to arrange it for you. Classes are available free under the NHS, but not nationwide as yet, so it will all depend on where you live. However, these classes are not suitable for those whose problems arise from aggressive outbursts nor for those loudmouthed people who are too fond of speaking their mind out of turn.

COUNSELLING

If you find your behaviour difficult to understand it may be wise to discuss it with a counsellor, who will be able to help you handle your own personal life better. We are all different and what helps one person does not necessarily help others. There are times when individual help is needed. Counsellors are also all different, use different techniques and come from different backgrounds, so you need to find one in whom you feel you can confide and with whom you feel comfortable. Make sure that your counsellor understands the mood changes which occur because of PMS, and takes them into account. It is wise to ensure that the first interview takes place during your 'good', postmenstrual phase, when you are more likely to be able to give an accurate account of the behavioural changes you experience monthly.

Abnormal behaviour in the premenstruum may be difficult to live with once normality has returned. Episodes like throwing away a good job, assaulting your nearest and dearest, shouting at neighbours or going on an expensive shopping spree may bring new problems to be faced after menstruation. Counselling may be particularly useful in helping to resolve some of the guilt resulting from such abnormal behaviour in the premenstruum.

If your problem is causing marital or relationship problems you may be better seeking the advice of a Relate Counsellor (they used to be called Marriage Guidance Counsellors), while if your problems have been worse since the loss of one near and dear to you a bereavement counsellor may be more suitable.

Psychotherapy
is an old and extremely respectable branch of medicine, but it is of doubtful value in treating a disease such as PMS which has a hormonal basis. It may help a woman to understand her mood swings and how to cope with them, and also relieve the guilt which may result from her PMS actions. The types of psycho-

logical treatment likely to be helpful are counselling, cognitive therapy and behaviour therapy.

Cognitive Therapy

aims to teach the patient to alter modes of thinking which aggravate or prolong anxiety. For instance, anxious patients often have palpitations or momentary giddiness, which they fear might be the beginnings of a heart attack or stroke. By altering such beliefs therapy can help to reduce anxiety.

Behavioural Therapy

attempts to teach patients how to get rid of unhelpful ways of coping, such as running away from situations which might cause anxiety, and replace these with useful and helpful ways of thinking; thus the patient will gradually face up to her own particular phobias.

HYPNOSIS

Hypnosis is the production of an artificial sleep in which the individual appears to be in a deep sleep without any power to change his or her mental or physical condition, except under the influence of external suggestion or direction by the hypnotist. When the subject 'wakes up' again, he or she has no conscious memory of what he or she has done or said while in the hypnotic state. It may be helpful in certain specific instances, such as trying to stop smoking or abusing alcohol, the relief of chronic pain and in overcoming phobias. It can be used to ease pain, and some dentists achieve painless removal of teeth under hypnosis. If pain in a limited area of your body occurs premenstrually, then hypnosis may possibly prove beneficial but, so far as I know, no successful way has ever been found to use hypnosis to correct the many different hormonal problems which come with PMS.

Self-hypnosis

This has been advocated by Duncan McColl (among others), who has produced a PMS tape which blends self-hypnosis, positive suggestion and professional advice. It is suggested that you play the tape every night at bedtime for three months, so that the positive suggestions sink in during natural sleep. It is claimed that it not only relieves PMS but any accompanying period pains as well, but there is only anecdotal evidence that it works.

ACUPUNCTURE

This ancient Chinese treatment uses accurately-placed needles to stimulate areas which are responsible for the health of particular organs of the body. This can be very valuable in certain localized disorders, especially the relief of pain. It is frequently used very effectively as an anaesthetic for dental extractions and in China they use it for more major operations, such as the removal of a lung. It is sometimes successful in relieving the pain of migraine and backaches, although several courses of treatment may be necessary. In some areas of Britain it is available on the NHS. It does not cope with the cause of recurrent pain which comes back during each cycle in the premenstruum, and is of less value in curing the psychological symptoms of PMS.

AROMATHERAPY

When you're feeling low, unloved and desperate, what could be nicer than being spoiled by having a gentle massage with fragrant oils? It is certainly relaxing and beneficial in easing stress and tension, whatever the cause, be it PMS, menstrual magnification or unrelated to menstruation. Aromatherapists emphasize the therapeutic qualities of the oils, which, they say, contain substances essential for the proper working of the body, and especially the brain. They also differentiate therapeutic oils from the fragrant perfume oils.

Although there is a lot of talk about absorption through the skin of the various essential oils required for the healthy functioning of the body, there is no evidence to support the suggestion that any significant amount of these oils does actually get absorbed into the bloodstream, where they are supposed to alter the body's metabolism or chemistry. The oils would have to pass through the upper corny layer of the skin, into the dermis and subcutaneous tissue under the skin and be absorbed by fat cells and capillaries to pass into the bloodstream in an amount large enough and for long enough to alter the body's metabolism or brain chemistry. Some chemicals can be absorbed through the skin and are available as patches to ensure a prolonged action, such as with oestrogen for the menopause, in which the patches are kept on for three days. Patches containing triglycerine nitrate for angina sufferers are kept on for 24 hours. If the therapeutic oils really had this marked effect and were absorbed into the blood, altering brain chemistry, then they would have to be licensed by the Committee of Safety of Medicine.

There are also aromatic oils which you can use when relaxing in the bath, and oils you can use to massage your abdomen and back. So, use aromatherapy to relax yourself, if you find it effective, but don't expect it to get to the root of your PMS.

OSTEOPATHY

For almost 100 years, osteopaths have believed that most diseases result from minor deformation of the spinal column, which they believe has bad effects on the nerves, cerebrospinal fluid and blood vessels. The idea is that gentle manipulation will cure these problems. It is true that manipulation of the spine will help certain types of backache and shoulder pain, and cranial osteopathy is often very helpful with some types of migraine, especially in patients who have a history of a whiplash injury to the neck. If your premenstrual symptoms are limited to just bone pains, then osteopathy may prove beneficial.

Reflexology
is the ancient Chinese art of foot massage. The reflexologist gently massages and presses the soles of the feet to stimulate the energy paths to various parts of the body linking the vital organs. This is pleasant and temporarily relaxing, but just how it helps your PMS symptoms is for you to find out: there have not been any trials, nor are any contemplated.

HOMOEOPATHY

Homoeopathy is the treatment of symptoms, not of disease states. It is based on the principle that if a herb or plant which, taken in excess, produces symptoms, then those symptoms are best relieved by giving that same herb but in a greatly reduced dilution. In short, it is treating like with like, as the name in its original Greek suggests.

Homoeopathy was started 200 years ago, before the discovery of bacteria and of hormones, when the fever of malaria was treated with quinine and syphilis was treated with arsenic. Dilutions of quinine, arsenic and numerous other herbs have been made; according to homoeopaths, the more they are diluted and shaken up, the greater their efficacy. The dilutions are so great that they cannot be called drugs and are known instead as 'remedies'. Homoeopathic treatment is available in Britain under the NHS in a few hospitals and by some general practitioners who have had additional training in homoeopathy. The remedies are also available in pharmacies over the counter and are relatively inexpensive.

Trials on farm animals by homoeopathic vets are said to have succeeded, and animals are not likely to understand what's going on in such a way that the placebo effect would come into play. We need to see these trials repeated by different researchers before we can be sure. In any case it does not always do to dismiss everything which science cannot explain. Homeopathy has its followers, and some of their remedies do ease symptoms, particularly anxiety and tension. As a medical doctor I do still tend to rely on science for my understanding of the world about me and I'm apt to be very sceptical about anything with which science cannot cope, but I would not reject out of hand any method that women might find helpful.

SOME LESS HELPFUL IDEAS

I recently took some books on alternative remedies out of the library, and was amazed to read of some of the things people will do in the name of health. The practices of 'urine therapy', for example, include pouring urine over open wounds. If you don't mind, we'll pass over this and also over art therapy, Bach flower remedies, bioenergetics, dance therapy, Kirlian photography, rebirthing, Rolfing, Shiatsu and the Silva method, all of which might, at best, perhaps improve the 'Feel-Well' factor.

Chapter 8

OVER-THE-COUNTER
MEDICINES

ARE THEY ANY USE?

Very few of the over-the-counter remedies sold as PMS cures have any value at all. Some can even be dangerous. In Great Britain there is a government body called the Committee for Safety of Medicines which licenses all drugs and places all new ones into various categories, including those which are safe enough to be sold by pharmacists in chemist's shops, commonly known as 'over-the-counter' drugs (OTCs), and those drugs which may only be obtained on a doctor's prescription. Before a new drug is licensed the manufacturer must produce evidence to the Committee that it has been fully tested on healthy human volunteers and on at least two different species of animals, and proved to have no side effects. The maker must also prove that the drug works, by subjecting it to clinical trials which show that it benefits patients with the disease(s) which it is claimed to help. Only then is a licence granted for doctors to use the new drug for the named disease(s).

A general practitioner may only write an NHS prescription for a drug which has been licensed by the Committee for Safety of Medicines. However, the Committee for Safety of Medicines does not look into the safety or effectiveness of vitamin or mineral preparations; these come under the scrutiny of the Ministry of Food and Agriculture which is concerned with the purity and safety of food products but not with their potential to produce or cure disease. For instance, it was the Ministry of Agriculture and Food which was involved in the epidemic of salmonella resulting from infected eggs in the late 1980s. In this chapter we shall see that many so-called remedies for PMS can be sold over the counter because they come under the heading of foods, and that they would certainly not be licensed by the

Committee for Safety of Medicines if they were classed as drugs.

Thus it is through what amounts to a loophole in the law that the public spends £175 million each year on 'medicines' that are of little or no value. The regulations should be changed but the amount of money involved makes for powerful opposition to any such change. The dangers involved with vitamin B_6 (see below), for example, are now proved beyond any doubt.

Developing a major new drug and testing it to the extent required by the Committee for Safety of Medicines costs, on average, £120 million. Small wonder that some small companies see richer pickings to be had in the 'alternative' and 'herbal' markets.

VITAMINS AND MINERALS

Vitamins are vital, naturally occurring chemicals which are required by the body in minute quantities and are essential for normal growth and health. Our diet must contain vitamins and certain minerals for good health, but these vitamins and minerals are only needed in very, very small amounts and are contained in carbohydrates, fats and proteins. In animal experiments in the laboratory it is easy enough to devise diets for caged animals which are deficient in just one essential vitamin or mineral, and then to study the effect of the resulting deficiency disease. However in the case of humans it is quite different, and it is very difficult or even impossible to devise a diet deficient in only one vitamin or mineral. People who have a poor diet usually are deficient in several vitamins and minerals, as well as either proteins, carbohydrates or fats. Furthermore, the effects of poor nutrition take time to show and will be occurring throughout the month and not just before menstruation, so vitamin or mineral deficiency alone cannot account for PMS.

I am not claiming that vitamin deficiencies don't cause illness, as they certainly do: lack of vitamin C causes scurvy, lack of vitamin D causes rickets and so on, but in modern Britain these diseases rarely occur, since the very small amounts of vitamins which we need for good health are naturally found in our diets. What is more, the fact that lack of a certain vitamin causes one specific disease does not mean that you can blame it for any other sort of illness.

On the other hand, PMS affects well over a million women in Britain. We've seen the figure quoted as 10 million, but that's probably a bit steep if you consider that there are only about 30 million females in the country, counting all age groups. Add some six million women in the US, let alone the rest of the world, and you can hardly be surprised at the number of untried or 'harmless' pills and potions for PMS on the market. Information on the importance of adequate vitamins in the diet is contained regularly in women's weekly and monthly journals. In 1991 the *Ladycare 2000 Report* surveyed 650 women and noted that health issues were considered the most important, with 87 per cent agreeing that vitamins and minerals were essential to good health. I have also read that a major national chain of chemist's had some 175 such 'health' products on sale; when I went to look, that figure seemed to be not far wrong.

Doctors have long known that vitamins A, D and E can be harmful or even fatal in large amounts; for example, there is a well-documented case of polar explorers dying from vitamin D poisoning because they ate too much polar bear liver. Even a very small excess of vitamin D can be dangerous. The amount of each vitamin needed for good health is generally only a few milligrams daily. (A milligram, or mg, is about the weight of one grain of sugar; there are 28,000 mg in an ounce.) Some vitamins (D, for instance,) are only needed in micrograms (mcg) – a microgram is one thousandth of a milligram.

Doctors traditionally divide the vitamins into two types: A, D and E are the 'fat-soluble' vitamins – they dissolve in fat but not in water, so the body cannot get rid of them quickly and they build up in the tissues. Vitamin C and all the many B-complex vitamins were once thought to be completely harmless, even in huge quantities, because they dissolve in water and so any excess is quickly excreted in the urine. However, we now know that at least some of the water-soluble vitamins can cause serious problems if taken in excess.

When I am asked about vitamins and PMS – and I very often am, of course – I usually use the analogy of oil and the car engine. Car engines need oil, and any mechanic will tell you that if you lost all your oil the engine would be wrecked in seconds.

Now, some people might think that because one gallon of oil is vital, two or three gallons must surely be better, so they should run off to the garage for another couple of cans and pour it all in. In fact, even a smallish excess of oil may well get onto your clutch and make it slip; if you filled the engine full up to the top you would never get it started (though you might do an awful lot of damage if you tried). Vitamins are like that: you need enough, but too much may cause problems.

Let's now take a close look at the various vitamins and minerals which are often claimed to help with PMS.

Vitamin B$_6$ (Pyridoxine)

Vitamin B$_6$, known by its chemical name 'pyridoxine', is the first on the list of over-the-counter preparations which we will consider, not only because it is so frequently advised for PMS but because of the serious harm it can cause. Schaumberg and his colleagues in New York were the first to report (in the *New England Journal of Medicine* in 1983) on seven cases, some wheelchair-bound, with severe nerve damage that had been caused by excessive doses of vitamin B$_6$. Schaumberg, a neurologist, had earlier studied the nerves of dogs and rodents when trying to find a cure for peripheral neuritis (a chronic and painful nerve disease, especially common among diabetics and alcoholics). Schaumberg showed by microscopic studies of nerve endings that an overdose of vitamin B$_6$ given to dogs and rodents caused the same abnormalities, with the same degeneration of peripheral nerve endings as are seen in biopsy specimens of nerves in humans who suffer from peripheral neuritis.

There have since been several studies to confirm the harmful effects of vitamin B$_6$, including a study on 'The Characteristics of Pyridoxine Overdose Neuropathy Syndrome' which I co-authored with my son Dr Michael Dalton in 1987 and which won the Cullen Nutrition Prize at the Royal Free Hospital, London. This showed that among 172 women taking vitamin B$_6$ and with a high pyridoxine blood level 60 per cent already had signs of nerve damage. The damage occurred after taking the vitamin for six months or more, either continually or inter-mittently, and the duration was more important than the actual

VITAMIN B6 POISONING

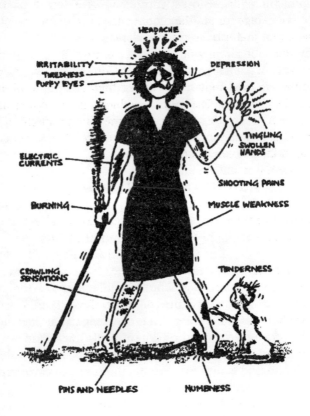

Figure 28: Symptoms of vitamin B₆ overdose

dosage. Symptoms of nerve damage were pins and needles in the arms and legs, areas of numbness, supersensitivity or burning of the skin, muscle weakness and general itching (Figure 28).

In 1990, Doctors Kleinjen, ter Riet and Knipschild in the Netherlands did a further study of all the published controlled trials in which B_6 had been used as treatment for PMS, and they found no evidence that it had any beneficial effect.

PMS sufferers must understand the dangers of taking extra vitamin B_6, and realize that there is no evidence whatsoever that a deficiency of it causes PMS. Vitamin B_6 is present in most foods, particularly cereals (especially wholegrain), egg yolk, fish, meat, chicken, liver, kidneys, dried yeast, bananas and avocados. It is only required in a minute quantity, no more than 2 to 4 mg daily (the RDA, or recommended daily allowance) – about the same weight as 2 to 4 grains of sugar.

People on a good normal diet will take in this amount in their first spoonful of cereal or quarter slice of toast at breakfast, although the gut will not normally absorb more from food than is required by the body. The problem which many women have with vitamin B_6 overdose seems to be some kind of 'hitch' in the body's mechanism for excreting this water-soluble vitamin. If they stop taking extra vitamin B_6, their symptoms usually disappear within a few months, but there may be permanent damage if excessively large doses have been taken. However, even those women whose B_6 overdose symptoms seem to have disappeared after they have stopped taking B_6 will get their nerve symptoms back after months or even years if they start taking B_6 again.

Some people have claimed that no damage will occur if vitamin B_6 is taken together with other vitamins of the B-complex group, or together with other vitamins or minerals, but there is no justification for this claim. Microscopic examinations of affected nerves in humans, dogs and rats does not support the idea – B_6 is dangerous no matter what you take it with.

**VITAMIN B_6 IS THE ONE OPTION
FOR TREATMENT FOR PMS
WHICH SHOULD BE
POSITIVELY AVOIDED.**

Vitamin E

A recent three-month trial at a medical school in the US showed that the various psychological symptoms of PMS were reduced by 27 per cent and physical symptoms by 38 per cent in women who took 400 IU (international unit) of vitamin E, compared with those taking a placebo, who only showed a 14 per cent reduction in physical symptoms and no change in emotional symptoms. The study found the natural vitamin more effective than the synthetic variety.

It is important to bear in mind that PMS has a high 'placebo response' and that the results of such trials often disagree with each other, partly because PMS symptoms are hard to pin down and measure accurately. This is the first trial of this vitamin for PMS; there will need to be more clinical trials before the effect of vitamin E is accepted, but this one is a move in the right direction. Vitamin E will certainly not do any harm, but it is not needed by anyone having a good, varied diet.

Multivitamin Preparations

It has been claimed that one in every three of Britain's adults takes some kind of vitamin supplement daily. In the majority of cases this is at best a waste of money, at worst it is dangerous. Different women have different dietary habits, especially in a multicultural nation like ours, and that includes PMS sufferers. If you are eating a good, varied diet then there is no need for extra vitamins or minerals. If you feel your diet is poor, then it is more important to change your diet to a healthy one, be it British, Italian, Greek or Chinese. A poor diet will in the end lead to poor health and to deficiency diseases which cause symptoms throughout the month and not just premenstrually. But even a very poor diet is unlikely to be deficient in all the vital vitamins and all the trace minerals, so even if you did have to take an artificial supplement, what would be needed would be a 'tailor-made' pill to correct your personal deficiencies rather than the 'shotgun' approach of taking a supplement containing every vitamin and mineral. Unless you are in a most unusual situation, such as being a polar explorer or an astronaut, you don't need any supplement, just a good diet. During the Second World War, because of the shortage of imported butter, oranges and lemons, expectant mothers and children received free vitamin tablets which contained vitamins A, C and D (but please note not any vitamin B and no multivitamins).

A good, varied diet need not be any more expensive than a bad one, and may well be cheaper. It's also likely to be more interesting. The starchy foods recommended to be taken every three hours for PMS (Chapter 6) are among the cheapest of ingredients.

If you have any doubts, I would suggest reading *The Premenstrual Syndrome Special Diet Cookbook* by Jill Davies, published in 1991.

I once sent my secretary into a branch of a well-known health store, asking her to seek out the manager and tell him or her that she suffered from PMS. She was not asked any questions at all about her diet or her PMS, but she emerged carrying six different bottles of vitamins and mineral supplements, with no instructions on their use and minus a sum of money that equalled her weekly salary. Does this help to explain why the vitamin and mineral supplement market was valued in 1990 at £175 million, with the figure rising annually?

Magnesium and Zinc

The human body only requires minute traces of the metals magnesium and zinc to function normally, and there is no extra benefit when the amount is increased. Such traces are required by both sexes and by women at all times of the menstrual cycle; there are no studies to suggest that women require more magnesium or zinc than men, or that they need more at any particular time of the month. The studies done in the US by Dr Guy Abraham centred on menstrual distress and *not* PMS.

Again, people who are on a good, healthy, varied diet need have no fear of a deficiency of trace minerals. The best sources of magnesium are:

- cereals
- green vegetables
- fruit
- seafood
- nuts.

Zinc is present in:

- milk
- vegetables
- meat
- fish
- sunflower seeds.

I'll say it again: if your diet is poor, it is better to think about your *whole* diet rather than guess about whether there might be some particular deficiency to be fixed with a tablet.

Magnesium OK is a food supplement which is drug-free but contains seven trace minerals and six vitamins *including vitamin B_6*. If you really must start on it, or on anything like it, keep an eye open for any of the nerve problems which may result from taking Vitamin B_6. Far simpler – and cheaper – would be not to take it at all.

One must be very careful about metals in general. Lead (chemically similar to zinc) has long been known to be a poison, and so are arsenic, beryllium, mercury and plutonium. It is now thought that aluminium may be involved in Alzheimer's disease. A controversial alternative remedy for Multiple Sclerosis is chromium, but in 1993 a woman died after taking large amounts of chromium orotate. The inquest into the cause of her death returned an open verdict, but the coroner said: 'there must now be a question-mark against chromium.'

It is often a question of quantity – sodium and potassium, for instance, are absolutely vital for key processes in the body, but a large excess of either will kill. Phosphorus, another metal needed for strong bones, produced a ghastly disease called 'phossy jaw' in workers producing matches in the last century. Just as in the hatmaking industry, where mercury poisoning caused madness, hence the phrase 'mad as a hatter'.

Iron

Iron is another metal which a healthy body requires and which may be at too low a level if the diet is poor. There are some individuals who do have difficulty in extracting sufficient iron from their food, even if they take in a good diet with plenty of fresh vegetables, fruit, eggs, kidney and liver. These people are advised to have regular courses of iron, but this has nothing to do with PMS.

Iron deficiency results in anaemia. Other causes of anaemia are increased blood loss through heavy menstruation, bleeding gums or haemorrhoids. Anaemia will cause symptoms throughout the month, including tiredness and lack of stamina, which will be more noticeable in the premenstruum. A simple blood test will detect anaemia, and if it is present iron therapy will help while the cause of the anaemia is being corrected. There are many types of iron tablets available from chemists, without prescription, but iron tablets do have different effects on different women. In some they cause constipation and in others they result in diarrhoea, so if you do have difficulty with one type, speak to the pharmacist who may help you choose another sort.

Calcium

Calcium is often added to multimineral preparations designed to help PMS. It is an important mineral and a lack of it can cause peridontal (gum and tooth) disease, hypertension (high blood pressure) and osteoporosis (brittle bones – most common in women after the menopause), but is of no special benefit to PMS sufferers. However, women considering their diet would be wise to ensure that they are getting enough calcium now, in their menstruating years, to prevent osteoporosis from occurring after the menopause. This applies particularly in those women whose mothers had a 'dowager's hump' or fractures of the wrist or hips, since osteoporosis tends to run in families.

Since the Second World War, all white bread sold in the UK must by law contain added calcium. White bread is therefore a very rich source of this mineral, containing twice as much as brown bread. The present fashion for eating wholemeal bread to increase the high fibre content of the diet may therefore be the cause of future trouble for many women unless they look elsewhere for extra calcium. Calcium is also present in milk, cheese, fish, watercress and many vegetables.

NATURE'S PLANTS
Oil of Evening Primrose

Oil of Evening Primrose contains one of the essential fatty acids, *gamma linoleic acid*, which is required by the brain cells for their proper functioning. Again, the essential fatty acids are required equally by men and women and at all times of the menstrual cycle, so they have no place in the treatment of PMS. They are, however, thought to be helpful for both sexes in the treatment of atopic eczema, and have been passed by the Committee of Safety of Medicines for atopic eczema and breast tenderness, but not for PMS (or anything else). It is reported the US Food and Drug Administration have banned Oil of Evening Primrose as it has not proved effective.

In 1993 Aila Collins and colleagues in Sweden carried out a well-designed double-blind controlled study reported in *Obstetrics and Gynaecology* on the use of high-dose Oil of Evening Primrose in PMS. Their study concluded: 'Treatment with essential fatty acids is ineffective therapy for PMS.' Such improvement as did occur was the same while receiving placebo or active medication, and they attributed this to 'either the placebo effect or participation in the study'. This confirmed the findings of a similar trial by Drs Khoo, Munro and Battistutta in Australia in 1990.

Furthermore, in June 1993 Drs J. Berth-Jones and R. A. C. Graham-Brown, both dermatologists at the Royal Leicester Hospital, reported in the *Lancet* on placebo-controlled trials on essential fatty acid supplementation in atopic dermatitis and reported 'no effect from medication'. This confirmed the findings in previous trials by dermatologists Bamford and his team in 1985, and Rilliet and his team in 1988.

The data-sheet giving prescribing information to doctors advises special precautions in prescribing Oil of Evening Primrose to epileptics.

Starflower oil is another such 'remedy' which has recently been introduced. It is claimed to have the same effect as Oil of Evening Primrose. Enough said.

Herbal Preparations

Some drugs, such as opium, cocaine or digitalis, are derived from herbs or plants and can be dangerous if used by the public without medical knowledge. Digitalis, for instance, has a powerful effect on the heart: it can be a life-saver when used properly, a killer if misused. It is found in the common foxglove in your garden. Such herbs are subject to licensing by the Committee of Safety of Medicines. Many other herbs, which have only mild actions, are not subject to the scrutiny of the Committee but the Medicines Control Agency does issue product licences for about 200 herbal products, which have 'PL' on their label and may be sold as medicines.

Other products may be sold freely from shops and health stores and prescribed by herbalists and nutritionists. Manufacturers of such preparations do not have to reveal the contents or the dosages, which they can change whenever they like. No trials are necessary before marketing such products; many people think they should be. For instance, there is a new herbal food supplement designed to alleviate PMS symptoms called *PM Comfort* which is sprayed under the tongue for at least seven or 10 days before menstruation is due. It is claimed that the natural (but secret) herbs benefit the female reproductive and nervous systems and that effectiveness increases with use. I know of no trials which support these claims, and since the formula is secret I can't comment on the effects of any of the ingredients. I have even seen a product which states more openly that it 'seems' to benefit PMS. You can be sure that any product which 'seems' to be of benefit has not been subjected to any trials to test its value.

The actions of certain herbs are mild and soothing and may be useful in removing some, but not all, symptoms of PMS. They include mild analgesics for the relief of pain, hypnotics to induce sleep, tranquillizers to ease tension and diuretics to increase urine output. The plant *Agnus castus* is often used for PMS and is claimed to have a balancing effect on hormones, regulating blood sugar, reducing salt intake and correcting nutritional deficiencies. *Pulsatilla* is recommended for sensitive women who tend to get weepy, sad and pale premenstrually. *Motherwort*, *Passiflora* and *Skullcap* ease anxiety and stress, and *dandelion*, *bladderwort*, *ground ivy*, *burdock root* and *parsley* all help combat water retention. *Meadowsweet*, which contains the salicylates found in aspirin, is helpful for headaches and bone pains, while *feverfew* is a favourite for migraine sufferers.

The trouble with the unlicensed herbal preparations (no 'PL' on the packet) is that you probably can't be sure how much of the active ingredient you're getting, and it may vary from packet to packet. Neither do you necessarily know about any side effects which the active ingredient may have, or whether other active substances have found their way into the preparation. The best advice is to scrutinize the packet and, if the ingredients are not precisely stated, to avoid buying it.

An even more dangerous practice is picking your own herbs. Are you sure you can identify the plant? What may be the side effects, and how can you control the dosage? I need hardly point out that anyone without special knowledge who plays around with eating unknown plants may well end up very ill indeed.

Royal Jelly

Royal jelly is a substance which bees feed to a larva if they want it to hatch out as a queen; without it the same larva will turn into an ordinary worker bee. It has nothing to do with the British Royal Family, but you can see the attraction – some people might reason that anything that can turn a grub into a queen bee must be very special. Of course, this is no reason why the stuff should have any effect on human beings at all, let alone why it should cure PMS.

Interestingly, one of those TV consumer watchdog programmes recently claimed that more 'royal jelly' is sold in Britain than all the bees in the world could produce. I am not surprised.

Royal jelly does not require labelling, so it is anyone's guess what a particular product contains. It is claimed to be good for the blood and skin, and has also, more cynically but no doubt more accurately, been described as 'a very expensive type of sugar'. The Consumers Association magazine *Which? Way to Health* noted that royal jelly, believed by some to be a magical tonic, a panacea and an important dietary supplement was in fact a poor source of vitamins and minerals and no better than a helping of cornflakes. After all, a bowl of cornflakes would contain 30 times more riboflavin (vitamin B_2), 90 times more niacin (vitamin B_3), and 400 times more folic acid, and would be considerably cheaper than royal jelly, which can cost £35 per jar.

Ginseng

Ginseng is a plant whose use originated in Chinese medicine. It is widely advertised for its ability to rejuvenate women and claims to help eliminate toxins and help with stress. There is no evidence to support this, nor any information as to which symptoms are most likely to be relieved. There is no control over the contents of any particular preparation of ginseng, so they probably vary a great deal. There is no reason to believe that ginseng will rejuvenate women in their premenstruum, rather than throughout the whole cycle. Nevertheless there are always people who feel that any 'medicine' coming from the Far East must automatically be better than anything originating in the West. If it's mysterious it must be good, such people think.

Garlic Tablets

I have already mentioned (Chapter 3) that the manufacturers of garlic tablets have recently been advertising them as helpful for PMS without stating precisely which symptoms might benefit. Garlic is reputed to help lower blood pressure and reduce heart attacks. So we have yet another instance of the 'shotgun' approach – if a herb or a vitamin helps with such-and-such a problem, then why not claim that it is a remedy for other ailments, too?

CONCLUSION

As I said at the beginning of this chapter, very few of the over-the-counter remedies sold as PMS cures have any value at all, and some can be dangerous. The amount of money involved, however, makes for powerful opposition to any change in the regulations concerning such remedies. The dangers associated with vitamin B_6, for example, are now proved beyond any doubt, yet the stuff is still for sale everywhere.

So are cigarettes.

Chapter 9

DRUGS TO RELIEVE SYMPTOMS

There is a difference between finding something to relieve your symptoms and finding the cause of the symptoms, and then both relieving the symptoms and preventing their return. Take the example of headaches. You can get rid of these with aspirin or paracetamol, but taking the tablet will not prevent a return of the headache after a few hours, unless you can find the cause and deal with it. There are many different causes of headaches, including a bump on the head, a hangover, blocked sinuses when you have a cold, eyestrain, infections or a food allergy. If the cause of the headache is obvious and unlikely to return, such as a blow on the head, then simple relief of the symptoms is sufficient. But if the headaches keep returning it is wiser to search for the cause and get it remedied, as when the headaches are due to eyestrain, which can be corrected quite simply by wearing glasses.

This chapter deals with relieving symptoms with drugs, without searching for the cause, and contains many suggestions which will be helpful (while you are charting the precise timing of your symptoms) in discovering whether you really have PMS or menstrual distress (also known as menstrual magnification). It is also worthwhile starting the three-hourly starch diet at this time too (see Chapter 6).

Symptomatic treatment is aimed at relieving the most important symptoms, but PMS is a hormonal illness. One of the characteristics of all hormonal illnesses is that they produce numerous widespread complaints in different systems of the body. For instance, diabetes affects the digestive system, energy, eyes, heart, blood pressure and kidneys. Many of the sympto-matic treatments recommended in this chapter need a doctor's prescription, but some are obtainable over the counter. If symptoms keep returning it is always worth searching for the cause and remedying that.

(Please note that all brand names mentioned are those available in the UK. As brand names differ world-wide I have also given the 'official' name [e.g. fenoprofen, mefanamic acid, etc.] of each drug discussed.)

ANALGESICS

Analgesics are pain-relievers and are valuable where pain is the main symptom, so they are useful for headaches, joint pains and period pains. Analgesics include *aspirin, paracetamol* and *prostaglandin inhibitors*, otherwise known as *non-steroidal anti-inflammatory drugs (NSAIDs)*, as well as the stronger drugs for extreme pain which are only obtainable on a doctor's prescription, such as those containing *codeine, pethidine* and *morphia*.

As well as relieving pain, the NSAIDs also reduce inflammation and fever. NSAIDs include aspirin, as well as the stronger ones such as mefanamic acid (Ponstan), indomethacin (Indocid), ibuprofen (Brufen, Motrin, Nurofen), and fenoprofen (Progesic), naproxen (Synflex). NSAIDs tend to cause indigestion and heartburn, so they are sometimes also administered as suppositories or as sustained-release capsules (e.g. Brufen, Fenbid and Indocid).

Aspirin

Aspirin has its limitations and is not the ideal drug for many. Some women, particularly asthmatics, are allergic to aspirin; in others it causes bleeding of the stomach lining. Aspirin is often included in pain-relieving mixtures such as Equigesic (meprobamate with aspirin), Hypon (caffeine and codeine with aspirin) and Migravess (metaclopromide with aspirin), so if you are sensitive to aspirin it will always be necessary to look at the ingredients carefully. The effects of aspirin overdose are variable, and in some instances a fatal overdose or permanent kidney damage can occur with only a relatively few tablets. The director of a dialysis unit in the US attended a PMS doctors' course because he had noticed that many of his current patients were admitted with kidney failure following a premenstrual overdose of aspirin.

Paracetamol

This does not cause gastric bleeding like aspirin and there are considerably fewer women who are allergic to it. It should be the first drug tried to relieve any pain, but the dose should not exceed two 500 mg tablets every four hours with a maximum total of 12 a day. Even a relatively small overdose can be fatal. Paracetamol can be sold over the counter as, for example, Panadol, but it is often combined with a more powerful analgesic in prescription-only medications like Cafadol (with caffeine). Paracodol, Solpadol and Tylex are compounds containing paracetamol with codeine, while Distalgesic contains an opiate as well as paracetamol.

Prostaglandins

Prostaglandins are chemicals released by damaged cells. There is now as group of drugs known as prostaglandin inhibitors or NSAIDs (non-steroidal anti-inflammatory drugs) which are able to lessen the number of prostaglandins released. Many different types of prostaglandin have been identified, which are released from different types of cells in the body, and many types of prostaglandin have their own prostaglandin inhibitor. *Ibuprofen* is most effective for the relief of joint and bone pain and is available over the counter. Pain in the uterus is caused by the release of the prostaglandin F2alpha, and the drug which is most helpful for the relief of uterine pain or dysmenorrhoea is *mefanamic acid* (Ponstan), which is best taken about seven days before the expected start of bleeding. In addition to reducing the pain at menstruation, mefanamic acid also reduces the blood loss by about a quarter, so it is also useful when there is heavy menstrual bleeding.

ANTIDEPRESSANTS

Depression can occur in healthy and unhealthy people and is not

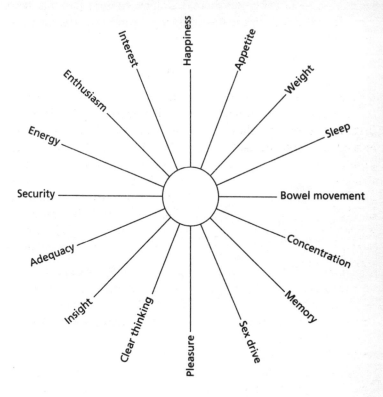

Figure 29: Depression is a disease of loss

necessarily a disease. It is healthy and natural to feel sad and depressed if your nearest and dearest dies suddenly, or if a fire devastates your house. It would be very unnatural if you did not show your emotions and were emotionally flat in such circumstances. Depression is also an illness when there is no real reason for the sadness, and when other faculties are affected. Depression is usually known by medical students as 'the disease of loss', for there is loss of sleep, loss of hope, loss of concentration, of security, of memory, of interests and enthusiasm, loss of regular bowel movement, of energy and a lot more besides (see Figure 29).

The depression which occurs with PMS is not the same as the typical, or common, depressive illness which psychiatrists and general practitioners so frequently have to deal with. In the 'typical' sort of depression there is usually a loss of appetite with loss of weight; in fact, the doctor may measure the improvement in a depressed patient by noting the increase in weight week by week. In PMS depression, things are quite different. There is often a craving for chocolates, sweets and the forbidden sugary foods, and there is a definite weight gain.

Although insomnia usually occurs in both kinds of depression, the types of sleep disturbance are very different. In normal depression the woman will get up in the early hours of the morning, perhaps make a cup of tea, read a book or even do some housework, and then doze until morning, but in PMS depression she never wants to get out of bed and would rather lie in until midday or later. Irritability is always present in PMS depression but not so in typical depression, when the patient may be too apathetic to be roused or annoyed. Whereas in typical depression there is a complete loss of interest in sex, the PMS sufferer, especially if she is a teenager, often feels an excessive sex urge, or even nymphomania, in the premenstruum. Men often find this extremely confusing – just when their partner is at her most awkward and nasty, she is more than usually interested in sex (see Table 4).

Table 4: Characteristics of Typical and PMS Depression		
	Typical	**PMS**
Appetite	loss	gain
Weight	loss	gain
Sleep	early waking	yearns for sleep
Irritability	sometimes	always
Sex interest	none	may be increased

Since depression is such a common symptom of PMS, there is always a temptation for a doctor to prescribe antidepressants rather than to consider the timing of the depressive symptoms and the fact that the depression comes and goes. This is especially so when the patient does not show the doctor her menstrual chart or fails to emphasize that her symptoms come before menstruation and that she feels fine afterwards. Premenstrual tension (PMT) includes depression, lethargy and irritability. The disadvantage of most antidepressants is that they cause drowsiness and so increase the tiredness which is already there, turning some patients into virtual zombies.

Triphasic Antidepressants

The *triphasic* antidepressants are the oldest, cheapest and easiest to use, and so they are usually the first sort a doctor will try. The group includes nortriptyline (Aventyl), clomipramine (Anafranil), amitriptyline (Tryptizol, Lentizol), imipramine (Tofranil), dothiapin (Prothiaden) and trimipramine (Surmontal), among others. They all need to be taken for about two weeks before their full effect is noticed. Some PMS patients may get panic attacks with triphasic antidepressants, and so the wise doctor will start them on a fairly low dose and only gradually increase it to a full dose if necessary. As these drugs cause drowsiness they are best taken at night, but they tend to lower one's sex drive. They also tend to cause a dry mouth and constipation. Figure 30 shows the type of antidepressant usually used for the different types of depression, but this is a speciality which belongs to the psychiatrists; all women are different in their symptoms and it is for specialists to determine the best type of medication for each patient.

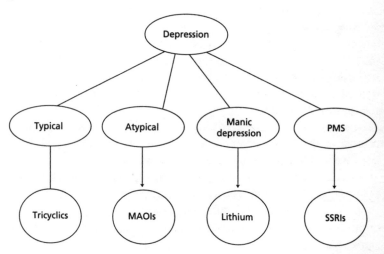

Figure 30: Antidepressants for types of depression

MAOIs

Monoamine oxidase inhibitors (MAOIs) are another group of antidepressants that do not take so long to work and are especially useful in atypical (non-typical) depressions such as occur with PMS. Two American doctors, Shader and Goldblatt, suggested the acronym 'TROUBLE' to describe patients most likely to benefit from MAOIs. It stands for:

T = Trouble
R = Regressive (going downhill)
O = Overanxious
U = Unstable
B = Bulimic
L = Labile (swinging up and down)
E = Episodic (good and bad times)

MAOIs work by preventing the build-up of too much of a chemical called *monoamine oxidase* in the brain cells. Many doctors and patients are not keen on using MAOIs because all sorts of food and drug restrictions are necessary: patients taking MAOIs must avoid cheese, meat extracts, red wine and be careful with the use of other drugs, especially ephedrine and amphetamine. The diet must be fully explained and understood by the patient and continued as long as MAOIs are used, since eating one of these 'forbidden' foods may cause a dangerous rise in blood pressure. If antidepressants are needed for PMS sufferers, then MAOIs are invariably more effective than the tricyclics, and may be given in spite of the annoying food restrictions. MAOIs often cause insomnia, so should be given early in the day; if necessary a hypnotic can also be taken at night to ensure sleep. Some preparations have an added tranquillizer, e.g. Parstelin, which is parnate plus stelazine.

Some of the common MAOI drugs are isocarboxazid (Marplan), phenelzine (Nardil) and tranylcypromine (Parnate).

In 1991, a team of molecular biochemists led by Zospan at the University of Chicago showed that progesterone works in the same way as MAOIs in inhibiting the accumulation of the enzyme monoamine oxidase in the brain. In short, they showed that in addition to its many other actions, progesterone is also a natural antidepressant. Fortunately progesterone, which is often given to PMS patients, does not require any dietary restrictions, even though it does act as a MAOI (Figure 30).

While MAOIs may help with premenstrual depression they will not help the other symptoms, in particular bloatedness and weight gain. In fact, in a short time there may be a remarkable gain in weight, but fortunately this disappears when the MAOIs are stopped. MAOIs are given continually throughout the cycle.

Lithium

Lithium is a trace element of which only a minute amount (or trace) is required by normal brain cells, but for some as yet unknown reason there are a few individuals of all ages and both sexes who sometimes require more than a trace. Lithium is particularly useful for those suffering from mania (being 'high') and manic depression, an illness in which there are unexpected short episodes of mania followed by longer episodes of depression. Sometimes such episodes start before menstruation, but more often they are unrelated to menstruation and last longer than 14 days. Lithium is sometimes useful in those patients who have depression throughout the cycle, becoming worse during the premenstruum, and in those with a family history of manic depression. Lithium is very effective in preventing recurrences, although the treatment does need to be long term, usually up to three years. As some people seem to absorb much more lithium than others it is important for the patient to be monitored with frequent blood tests to ensure that the amount of lithium in the blood does not reach a dangerous level (Figure 30). Patients are advised to maintain a good salt and water intake and to avoid dehydration. Lithium preparations available in the UK include Camcolit, Liskonum and Priadel (which is a slow-release preparation).

Serotonin-related Antidepressants

Medical science has recently reached a greater understanding of brain-cell chemistry in relation to a chemical called *serotonin*, which is a neurotransmitter. As early as 1984, Taylor, Matthew and Beng found that serotonin levels in blood platelets were low in PMS sufferers. This led to a new search for a drug which would prevent the loss of serotonin, known as the *Selective Serotonin Reuptake Inhibitors (SSRIs)*, which include *fluoxitine* (Prozac and Faverin), *paroxetine* (Seroxat) and *sertraline* (Lustral). These are proving especially helpful to sufferers of PMS, although they still need to be given throughout the cycle, whether the depression is present or not. They help with premenstrual depression and with the psychological symptoms, but not with the physical symptoms.

Patients should be started on a low dose to begin with, which is then gradually raised, and should not be given any within two weeks of receiving MAOIs and Beta blockers (see page 113). SSRIs are less likely to cause drowsiness than the tricyclics, but if they do, they should be taken at night.

Prozac has been the subject of a great deal of negative publicity in recent times. When Prozac was first used, too high doses were given and tragedies occurred. With lower doses, greater experience and better recognition of those most likely to respond, however, Prozac's results are most satisfactory.

TRANQUILLIZERS

Tranquillizers are given to patients with excessive anxiety, agitation, tension, irritability and insomnia, to calm them down. In the 1940s and 1950s barbiturates were used, until doctors realized that they were addictive and caused depression. They were replaced by a group of drugs called *benzodiazepines* (including valium, ativan, lorazepam, nitrazepam, flurazepam and temazepam) until they, too, were found to be addictive and to have unpleasant effects when stopped. Today no new patients should be started on benzodiazepines and those already on them are being gradually withdrawn under supervision.

If a sedative really is needed, there is another major group of tranquillizers including chlorpromazine, stelazine and sinequin, but they also need a prescription and require careful supervision. Some patients find that Beta blockers are effective tranquillizers (see page 113).

Hypnotics

Hypnotics are drugs which help you to sleep, but most of them are addictive and so should be used for a short time only. The commonest are the benzodiazepines, especially temazepam (Normison) and nitrazepam (Mogadon) but, as we have already noted, they are addictive, so if ever they are prescribed doctors are advised that the absolute limit is six weeks, whether taken continuously or for short spells. It is important to realize that the effect of even the short-acting benzodiazepines lasts longer than eight hours, so there is always some drowsiness for the first few hours the next morning.

Some herbal preparations are effective hypnotics and are not addictive; they should always be tried first before seeking a medical prescription. Camomile tea is claimed to be most effective if taken at bedtime.

Beta Blockers

Beta blockers are a group of drugs that act on the sympathetic nerves which control the involuntary muscles. These are not to be confused with the nerves which control our voluntary muscle movements such as those of our limbs and face, but there are internal involuntary muscles which we cannot control, including those of the heart, blood vessels and intestines. Beta blockers are valuable in the control of blood pressure, migraine and anxiety, and are often used to promote calmness and tranquillity in artists or musicians before a public performance. PMS sufferers may find them helpful to prevent panic attacks. They should be avoided by those with a history of asthma. Propranalol is the favourite form, which is present in Inderal and Tenormin.

DIURETICS

Diuretics are drugs which make the kidneys do more work, so that the output of urine is increased. Diuretics are temporarily effective in removing bloatedness, water retention, breast swelling, puffy eyes and swollen ankles, but they do not help the psychological symptoms of PMS and may well increase the

113

tiredness. The action of diuretics has been likened to bailing out water from a boat, instead of blocking up the hole and preventing the water getting in.

Diuretics are so effective that, all too often, although they are initially prescribed for use only in the premenstruum, women start taking them throughout the cycle, and then not just one tablet but two or three daily. The patients then demand even stronger diuretics. In short, diuretics are addictive, and any reduction of the dose must be done slowly, as otherwise there is such a drastic return of water retention that the patient will never again agree to stop taking them. It is now known that bloatedness is better controlled with a three-hourly starch diet (Chapter 6).

The early diuretic tablets tended to cause an upset of the sodium/potassium balance in the blood, resulting in a low blood potassium level, which causes exhaustion and muscle weakness. The newer diuretics are potassium-sparing and the side effects of low potassium are rarely seen, so it is no longer necessary to test the blood potassium level of patients taking diuretics. The common diuretics include ameloride (Midamore, Frumil, Kasoride), bumetanide (Burinex), frusimide (Frumil, Lasix), spironolactone (Aldactone) and thiazide (Aprinox, Hydrosaluric, Moduretic, Nordrex and Saluric).

INHALERS

Inhalers are valuable for women suffering from premenstrual asthma and nasal obstruction (blocked nose). They are so effective that although they are initially prescribed to be used only during the premenstruum or when an attack occurs, all too often they become a habit and get used daily or several times a day. Some inhalers contain adrenalin, which may increase the PMS mood swings, so it is worthwhile also keeping a chart of the number of times you use the inhaler, to find out whether the asthma really is menstrually related.

ANTICONVULSANTS

Anticonvulsant drugs are used to control epileptic fits. Even those sufferers who think their fits only occur in the premenstruum are advised to continue their anticonvulsant medication until the diagnosis of PMS is confirmed. When patients are well stabilized on the right dose of progesterone and the three-hourly starch diet, the doctor can start a reduction of the anticonvulsant therapy and, in many cases, finally stop the drug altogether.

PHYSICAL SYMPTOMS

PMS is not limited to psychological symptoms. There are twice as many physical symptoms, which tend to be treated by other departments of medicine such as by the dermatologists, chest physicians, urologists, neurologists, ophthalmologists, rheumatologists, otologists and gastroenterologists. In each of these departments the consultant will only see a very small proportion of patients with PMS, and so will tend to treat such patients in the same way as other patients with chronic or recurrent symptoms. It is therefore up to patients who think that their physical symptoms are limited to the premenstruum to bring with them a menstrual chart to enable the consultant to confirm the diagnosis of PMS and treat them appropriately. This is especially important when surgical operations are being considered, such as for nasal obstruction and sinusitis, backache and disc problems, cystitis and urethritis, and raised intraocular pressure in glaucoma. If such operations are undertaken in patients whose symptoms are caused by PMS, then the results are not likely to be so satisfactory. If possible always try to have operations planned to take place *after* menstruation, during the good phase of your cycle when recovery will be better.

Chapter 10

PROGESTERONE TREATMENT

This chapter deals with progesterone treatment. It is one of many hormone treatments for PMS, which can only be given by registered medical practitioners. I make no apology for devoting a whole chapter to progesterone therapy, as PMS is a progesterone-related disease and those who understand and use progesterone therapy for PMS appreciate the full benefit it brings.

One is always surprised at how many doctors of various specialities will not accept the use of progesterone, although in private conversation they will admit that they have never used it and do not understand its properties, how to use it or how to adjust the dose – indeed, all too often they do not know the difference between progesterone and the progestogens (man-made progesterone).

Furthermore, one cannot say that progesterone has failed in a patient with well-diagnosed PMS unless one has also tried progesterone injections, for it is known that 10 per cent of women cannot absorb enough progesterone by suppository or pessary to be effective. Other hormone treatments, which rely on stopping menstruation and ovulation while retaining monthly vaginal bleeding, are dealt with in Chapter 11.

A TEST FOR PMS?

The typical gynaecologist's way of trying to track down PMS tends to be the use of blood tests, hormonal estimations, ultrasound scans and surgical procedures such as a D & C or laparoscopy (see Chapter 12). Such gynaecological tests are routinely done for PMS, but they are of no value. For example, doctors who believe that PMS is all to do with progesterone may reasonably and logically decide to test their PMS patients for the amount of progesterone in the blood. The bad news is that there is no simple, straightforward connection between blood progesterone levels and presence or absence of PMS, so doctors trying to make the connection may well begin to doubt that PMS exists after all, or that progesterone has anything to do with it. You can't blame them. The problem in PMS lies with progesterone receptors (see Chapter 4) and we cannot yet estimate by means of a simple test the number of progesterone receptors at a particular site in the brain. Later in this chapter we shall see why such tests don't prove anything about PMS, so non-specialists can be excused for not yet having all this up-to-date information.

Is there *any* test for PMS? Well, you already know that the obvious way is simply to chart the symptoms, but it would be nice to have a blood test as well, because it could be done straight away in a hospital, without sending the patient home with nothing but a blank chart and instructions to come back in few months. It would also be handy in legal cases where the defendant claims PMS as a defence but has no menstrual chart. (One is perpetually amazed at top-ranking gynaecologists and even professors who do not ask their patients to keep a menstrual record of their symptoms or dates of menstruation, and assume that their verbal statements are always completely accurate and that the length of their cycle is always 28 days!)

In fact, such a test does exist: it is for *Sex-Hormone Binding Globulin*, or SHBG. The test can only be done in Britain, and only under special circumstances will the NHS pay for it. For the test to be reliable the blood must immediately be *centrifuged* (spun in a fast-moving drum) and stored frozen until tested; this makes it practically impossible for the general practitioner to take the blood sample. The woman must not have had any medication for the past seven days; this includes vitamins, laxatives and pain-killers. She must not have had any hormonal medication – this includes the Pill – for a month. The test will not be reliable if the woman is very overweight or unusually hairy, or if she has a thyroid or liver disease.

In any case, this blood test with all its problems is not as reliable as the simple chart in diagnosing PMS, so all in all the chart is normally going to be the best option. As noted above, however, the test may be useful in certain legal cases, to provide factual evidence.

As mentioned, there are not yet any tests available to estimate the number of progesterone receptors in sufferers and compare them with the number in normal women. Such a test would not only be useful to diagnose PMS, but would also teach us a lot about the disease. At the moment, however, such information can only be obtained from animals or post-mortem examinations.

PMS is a *progesterone-related disease* and is due to a problem with the *progesterone receptors*, or more specifically the binding of molecules of progesterone to progesterone receptors (see pages 49–54 in Chapter 4). When there is a specific blood test to show the presence or absence of progesterone receptor antibodies, or even progesterone receptors, we will more easily be able to recognize which patients have PMS without having to rely on at least two months' recording, and it will be easier to distinguish those who will benefit from progesterone therapy.

At present many researchers refer to clinical trials which have not shown progesterone to be beneficial, and state that the work on progesterone is 'anecdotal' (meaning 'coming from patients' stories') and not scientifically proven. It is as well to remind them that insulin has never been subjected to double-blind placebo controlled trials for the simple reason that it is impossible to devise a trial with one insulin dose and one set menu for sufferers of different ages, occupations and severity. The problem of clinical trials is considered separately in Chapter 14.

ISOLATING PROGESTERONE

Allen and Corner from the University of Rochester were the first to succeed in isolating 150 micrograms of progesterone from the corpus luteum of pigs' ovaries, and in producing the chemical formula. When they wanted to obtain a gram of progesterone for further work on the new hormone, they had to obtain 200 lb of pigs' ovaries from a slaughterhouse in Chicago. This explains the exorbitant price of progesterone in the early days. Later it was obtained from pregnant mares' serum (also abbreviated to

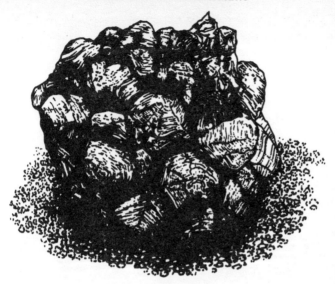

Figure 31: Elephant's toes

PMS!). In the late 1930s Russell Marker, a biochemistry student, worked out how it should be possible to synthesize progesterone from a chemical, 'diosgenin', found in certain plants, by altering the side-chain of the molecule.

Marker took a year off from university and searched the Central American jungle, where he found the black lumpy root of a yam called 'dioscorea', 'elephantipes' or 'elephant's toes', which contains diosgenin. Suddenly he was able to produce more than half of the current available world supply of progesterone, and the price of progesterone tumbled.

Nowadays, the progesterone in our suppositories and injections is synthesized from soya (Figure 32). Much of it is then converted into progestogens, cortisone, hydrocortisone, oestrogens and testosterone, for which there is a greater demand – thus making greater profit.

THE CLAUBERG TEST

Soon after the isolation of progesterone, research scientists showed that when female animals and women were given a

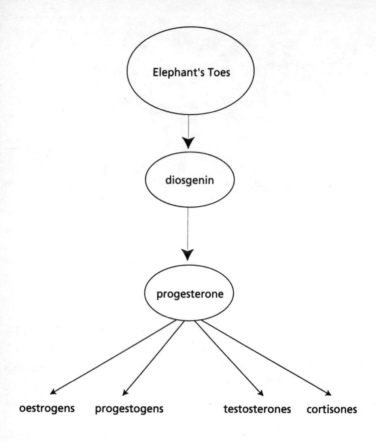

Figure 32: Production of progesterone

course of oestrogen and progesterone, vaginal bleeding occurred when the course ended. This ability to produce bleeding has been used in the *Clauberg Test*, in which drugs are tested and, if bleeding results, that drug is known as a *progestogen*. But although progestogens have this ability to produce *withdrawal bleeding*, in other ways they do not have exactly the same properties as natural progesterone. In particular, the blood progesterone level rises when progesterone is given, whereas if progestogens are given the blood progesterone level drops: exactly the opposite of what is required in PMS (Figure 33).

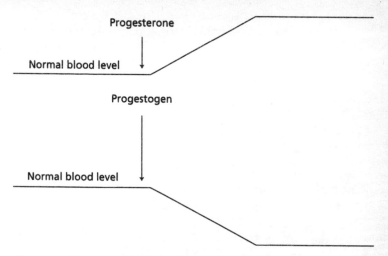

Figure 33: Effect of administration of progesterone and progestogens on blood progesterone level

RULES FOR PROGESTERONE TREATMENT

Progesterone treatment is used for:
- PMS
- *In vitro* fertilization
- Defective luteal phase (see Chapter 13)
- Habitual miscarriages
- Threatened miscarriage
- Morning sickness
- Pre-eclampsia
- Postnatal depression
- Menopause

For effective treatment there are certain general rules which must always be followed, regardless of the disease being treated. The first rule is that progesterone should be started *before* symptoms appear, because we know that once the symptoms are actually present, progesterone treatment is not effective. Another rule is that the sufferer *must* be following the three-hourly starch diet for at least one week before starting progesterone. Again, the dose must be sufficiently high to increase the level of the progesterone receptors. The final rule is that progesterone must be used *systemically* (by injection, by implant or through the vagina [pessaries] or the rectum [suppositories]). It cannot be given by mouth (see Chapter 11). The man-made progestogens can be given by mouth, which is so much easier, but since they make PMS worse, rather than curing it, it's no good indulging in wishful thinking. If the patient is suffering from thrush, this should be treated first.

Rules of progesterone treatment
- Use before symptoms start (prophylactic use)
- Blood sugar level must be stable
- High dose essential
- Oral administration is ineffective
- 10 per cent of women cannot absorb suppositories effectively
- Treat any thrush first

Now let's look at the rules listed above in more detail.

Prophylactic Use

Progesterone needs to be given before the symptoms appear, and is generally ineffective once symptoms have started. For PMS, progesterone should be given 14 days before the expected day of menstruation. In general this means starting on Day 14 if there is a 28-day menstrual cycle, but for those with a 24-day cycle the progesterone should be started on Day 10, or for those with a 32-day cycle it is started on Day 18 (see Figure 34).

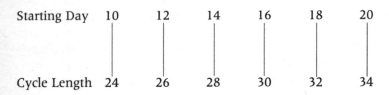

Starting Day	10	12	14	16	18	20
Cycle Length	24	26	28	30	32	34

Figure 34: Time of starting progesterone with different lengths of menstrual cycles

This again emphasizes the need for completing a menstrual chart before beginning progesterone treatment, as otherwise the whole exercise is based on guesswork and averages. If progesterone is started before ovulation, there may be bleeding at ovulation or after a few days; in short, it will cause menstrual irregularity. The time of starting is a problem in clinical trials, in which the protocol is likely to insist on all volunteers starting medication on a set day, usually Day 14 or 16, regardless of their own individual length of menstrual cycle which may be anything from 21 to 36 days (see Chapter 1, page 10).

Stable Blood Sugar Level

Chapter 4 discusses the reason for maintaining a steady blood sugar level, and Chapter 6 discusses how this can be best be achieved. The *three-hourly starch diet* (Chapter 6) means eating small portions of starchy food every three hours and within one hour after getting up and one hour or less before going to bed. This dietary regime is usually started at the same time as menstrual charting, and often brings sufficient relief so that progesterone treatment is no longer necessary – the doctor sends the patient home to keep a chart for some months and to try the diet, and by the next appointment she needs no further treatment.

High Dose

In Chapter 4 I discussed the work of Blaustein and his colleagues. In tests on animals, they showed that when the first dose of progesterone was effective, the second dose was not – even if double the amount was used there was no reaction. After the first dose, the animal became insensitive to small doses and now required some 40 times more to produce the same reaction. Experience has shown this also to be true when using progesterone on humans. Often there is some benefit from the first dose, but not after that, unless a very high dose is given. Generally speaking, suppositories of *400 mg used twice daily is the lowest effective dose* for cases of PMS which are not completely relieved by the three-hourly starch diet.

During pregnancy, the placenta produces up to 40 times the highest level of progesterone reached by a menstruating woman, (about seven days before menstruation starts; see Figure 11, page 24). Even with our very best methods of giving progesterone we cannot get anything like this much progesterone into the patient, so there is never any danger of overdose with progesterone. This means that a good supply of progesterone suppositories can safely be given to patients who have previously risked their lives by taking overdoses of antidepressants, tranquillizers or painkillers. *You cannot overdose on progesterone.* In practice, the highest daily dose which can be used for the 14 premenstrual days is one daily injection of 100 mg together with up to six 400 mg suppositories. If these doses are ineffective the diagnosis must be reconsidered to see if the problem really is PMS.

Avoid Oral Progesterone

When progesterone is given by mouth, it passes into the digestive tract and on into the liver. There are very many progesterone receptors in the liver; they quickly break down the progesterone molecules, but not in the same way as progesterone molecules are broken down in other cells in the body. The compounds, or *metabolites*, formed when progesterone is broken down in the liver, cause short-lived episodes of drowsiness and sleepiness: in other words, progesterone acts like a tranquillizer and a sleeping pill. This is in general a bad thing – if such drugs are needed it is safer to use ones whose strength and action we can predict. Anyway, if progesterone is used properly the need for such drugs will probably disappear. These metabolites may also act on the lining of the womb, resulting in vaginal bleeding. For these reasons we can say that progesterone given by mouth is *worse than useless* in PMS.

Oral progesterone is not available in Britain, although it is in France. In the US there are many pharmaceutical firms promoting oral *micronized* progesterone dissolved in various products to improve the absorption, but the breakdown in the liver still occurs so the problem of the metabolites remains. Numerous British patients have been given oral tablets, capsules, jelly or gum in trials, but they do not work anywhere near as well as suppositories.

Progesterone Suppositories

Both in Britain and in the US progesterone suppositories are the most widely used treatment for PMS. The suppositories can be inserted rectally or vaginally – in the latter case they should technically be known as 'pessaries'. In Britain, Cyclogest suppositories have been licensed by the Committee for Safety of Medicines and so can be prescribed on the NHS. Cyclogest is also available in Cyprus, Singapore and Hong Kong, and is currently being registered in Korea and South Africa.

In the US and many European countries, progesterone suppositories are made up by local pharmacies, but American pharmacy students are not even taught how to make up suppositories during their course of training. In Britain, because Cyclogest is licensed it is also quality controlled, which means that each suppository must contain the stated dose (400 mg or 200 mg), within a small margin. On a lecture tour to the US in 1985, progesterone suppositories were obtained from PMS Clinics in 14 different states. When these were analysed in Britain, only one contained within 3 per cent of the stated dose, indeed one suppository only contained 34 per cent! However, in the interval there has hopefully been an improvement in the quality of suppositories that can be obtained in the US.

There is a surprising difference in the absorption of progesterone by different women when progesterone blood levels are measured. So far no definite pattern has emerged, which means it is impossible to tell in advance whether a particular individual will need the minimum or even the maximum dose. The ideal dosage does not seem to be related to the severity of the PMS or to the type of symptoms. Nor does it seem to matter whether the progesterone is used rectally or vaginally; age, height and weight seem irrelevant, as do the number of pregnancies or miscarriages, previous pre-eclampsia, postnatal depression, contraceptive pill use or levels of the other menstrual hormones.

The medical records of over 1,000 PMS sufferers receiving progesterone, which were studied for the American Food and Drug Administration, showed that 10 per cent could not absorb adequate progesterone in the form of suppositories through the rectum or vagina, and needed the hormone in the form of injections. This means that nobody should say that progesterone doesn't work until injections have been tried for at least a month (see 'Progesterone Injections' below).

Because of the difference in the level of blood progesterone after using suppositories, it is difficult to determine an individual's optimum dose. It is still a matter of trial and error. After inserting a progesterone suppository, the rise in blood progesterone level never lasts as long as 24 hours; the average is 8 to 16 hours. This means that to maintain a constantly raised blood progesterone level, suppositories need to be used at least twice daily. The suppositories contain progesterone as a white crystalline powder dissolved in a mixture of waxes and fats designed to melt at body temperature. Two suppositories cannot usefully be inserted into the same orifice (vagina or rectum) at the same time, because there is then too much wax to allow the progesterone to penetrate through the membrane and into the bloodstream, resulting in less than a quarter of the dose being absorbed. It is possible, of course, to put in two suppositories at the same time, one in each place. In general, though, there is not a lot of point in this, as the body seems incapable of absorbing more than 400 mg of progesterone at any one time.

Using progesterone suppositories

- Use at least twice daily.
- Never insert two together.
- Never use tampon at time of insertion.

If suppositories are inserted rectally, the wax is eliminated in the faeces, whereas if inserted vaginally the wax comes away freely and some women complain of the mess. This can be avoided if a panty liner or sanitary towel is used at the time of insertion: 20 minutes later all the wax will have melted, so with a wash and a wipe any remaining wax and the panty liner can be removed. It is no good inserting a suppository at the same time as a tampon, because then the progesterone is absorbed by the tampon, not the body, and no benefit is obtained.

If suppositories are inserted rectally, then it is advisable to insert the blunt end first: this prevents any air entering and so avoids the flatulence and abdominal rumbling which some women notice after inserting a suppository rectally.

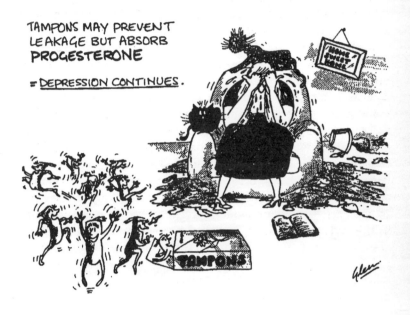

Figure 35: 'Happy tampons'

Progesterone Suspension

In the US, where Cyclogest suppositories are not available, the suppositories are made up locally by compounding pharmacists. Suppositories are difficult to produce because the base, or wax, must melt exactly at body temperature. If it has too high a melting point then some women will find them very gritty. If during manufacture the suppositories are heated too high or cooled too quickly, sharp crystals may form, which cause a pricking pain after insertion. Sometimes the base used causes irritation and diarrhoea. So, to overcome these problems in the US, progesterone is often sold in liquid form (as a liquid suspension), which is then inserted into the vagina or rectum using a blunt-ended syringe. Suspension has the added advantage of being cheaper. There is no demand for the suspension in Britain, although many British volunteers have acted as 'guinea pigs' to try it.

Thrush

Thrush (*candidiasis* or *moniliasis*) is a fungal infection of the vagina or mouth. Fungus should normally be present in the digestive tract; in fact it helps, together with millions of tiny bacteria, to digest our food. But when thrush gets outside the digestive tract it can cause problems. In the vagina it causes intense itching and a white flecky discharge, which is normally transmitted to the partner during sexual intercourse. If thrush is present when progesterone is used there will be an increase in the thrush symptoms, so the thrush should be treated first. The patient and her partner need only take one 150 mg capsule of fluconazole (UK brand name Diflucan) and within a few days the problem will be over. Alternatively the woman can use Canestan pessaries, which are obtainable over the counter, but she will be at risk of a recurrence if her partner is not treated simultaneously.

PROGESTERONE INJECTIONS

Progesterone given by injection causes a more reliable rise in blood progesterone level, so it is used initially in desperately severe cases when it is essential to get a quick result. There are some women who do not appear to benefit from as many as six suppositories daily but who get immediate relief with injections. Also, when patients are in hospital it is often easier for them to receive injections rather than suppositories. A few women who need daily supervision during the premenstruum because of suicidal or criminal tendencies, are best treated at first by injections given by the district or practice nurse, who can thus keep a discreet eye on them at their dangerous times.

Progesterone is insoluble in water but can be dissolved in alcohol, ether, chloroform and various oils. In Britain the progesterone used in injections is dissolved in an oil, *ethyloleate*, whereas in the US *arachis oil* is frequently used. Occasionally the progesterone crystals separate out after prolonged standing or in the cold and you can see them lying at the bottom of the glass ampoule. Should this occur, the crystals can easily be re-dissolved by *slowly and gently* heating the ampoule.

Progesterone injections need to be given into the buttocks,

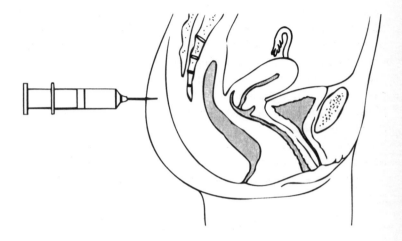

Figure 36: Site for progesterone injections

anywhere where there is a *one inch pinch of flesh*, but never in the thighs. Some are frightened of giving injections into the buttocks, fearing that they will touch the sciatic nerve. They need not worry – this nerve is safely hidden inside the pelvis and would need a six-inch needle and a hammer to reach it through the buttocks, but once the nerve reaches the thigh it is unprotected, so injections should not be given below the buttock fold (Figure 36).

The injection can be given by the practice nurse or district nurse, by the patient's partner or by the patient herself. Self-injections can be given while sitting down or while leaning the buttock against a table and then sliding the loaded syringe along the table (in this way it is bound to go in at right angles, as the flesh is held firmly by leaning on the table).

A survey in 1964 showed that half of the patients who were receiving progesterone injections were doing their own injections, and the proportion of patients managing their own injections appears to be about the same today. Women soon appreciate the advantage and time saved by not having to go down to the doctors' surgeries or wait in at home for the nurse. An added bonus is that they can have the injection just before their bath (as a spell in warm water helps disperse the oil).

Injections should be given on alternate sides of the buttocks. You could make a rule to use the left side on even dates and the right side on odd ones. Never inject into an area which is hot or sore. Soreness develops if the injections have been given in the same site and the oil has not had a chance to be absorbed by the nearby fat cells, which are clustered between muscle fibres. If the injections are being done at home, being given by the patient, her partner, mother or friend, they are best given before a bath, as mentioned above.

PROGESTERONE IMPLANTS

Pellets of pure progesterone implanted into the abdominal wall have brought from four to 12 months' relief to thousands of women over the last 40 years, and saved them from having daily injections or using frequent daily suppositories. Unfortunately, in 1991 the Committee for Safety of Medicines revoked the provisional licence for progesterone implants, asking the manufacturers to provide details of their safety, efficiency and pharmokinetics (the study of exactly how the drug is broken down in the body).

Unfortunately the manufacturers, Organon Ltd, did not consider it profitable to assemble all the required data and so closed down their production of progesterone implants. They also stopped production of their veterinary progesterone implants, which were used to prevent abortion in cattle. A search throughout the world has not yet found any other supplier of progesterone implants and the outlook is bleak. Organon did not stop making the oestrogen and testosterone implants used for the treatment of the menopause, as this is an ever-increasing market and highly profitable.

FOR HOW LONG?

The initial aim of progesterone therapy is to bring complete relief for at least three months, raising the dose at each consultation until relief is obtained. When there is no more suffering, the dose may be gradually reduced month by month. If the patient is receiving injections, these can be reduced to alternate days with suppositories on the non-injection days. If this is successful the doctor may try further reducing the dose by using an injection on one day in three, followed by two days on suppositories, and then gradually changing to suppositories only. In the same way, the number of suppositories being used can be gradually reduced, but never below two daily. At each consultation the dietary regime should also be discussed, for this is an essential part of progesterone treatment.

When one is on progesterone therapy menstruation may become scanty or stop completely. This should not be a cause for concern unless the patient is anxious to conceive. Progesterone is the pregnancy hormone, which appears in the blood after ovulation, and in the normal cycle if conception does not occur the progesterone level drops and menstruation takes place, which can be looked on as a failed pregnancy. Nature does not like repeated failures, and in the end the patient may stop ovulating. During pregnancy, menstruation and ovulation also stop for nine months, but no harm occurs.

If Nature had her way, women would be continually pregnant or breastfeeding. Thus they would have high progesterone levels all the time, with no menstruation for nine months every year or so for about 30 years. They would be having much higher blood progesterone levels for considerably longer than patients receiving progesterone therapy, so there is no need to fear any long-term side effects. In fact, a survey presented to the American Food and Drug Administration in 1983 (since published in this author's *Premenstrual Syndrome and Progesterone Therapy*; Heinemann, 2nd edn, 1984), included 15 PMS women who had been on continuous progesterone for more than 15 years. They were all well, free from symptoms and without any complications. Since then, the number of women who have been on progesterone continuously for 15 to 30 years has increased, but no unwanted side effects have been noted.

WILL I STILL NEED PROGESTERONE AFTER THE MENOPAUSE?

Generally women with PMS have an easy menopause. They recognize the menopause by the change in their menstrual pattern, with bleeding becoming lighter and happening less often, finally stopping altogether. Those receiving progesterone may not notice this happening and be free from the usual nasty menopausal symptoms such as hot flushes and night sweats. They are advised to continue with their normal dose of progesterone, using it continuously until there has been no menstruation for about a year, and then gradually reducing the dose month by month until there are no symptoms and no menstruation. It is only if the menopausal symptoms are severe and not relieved by progesterone that it is necessary to add some oestrogen. However if oestrogen is used then there must be regular bleeding to prevent the build-up of the lining of the womb. This means that the progesterone is stopped for a few days each month to allow vaginal bleeding.

When the menopause occurs the ovaries stop producing oestrogen, but other cells in the body take over the task of producing the special menopausal oestrogen called *oestrone*. Oestrone is produced from progesterone, but is not well absorbed when taken by mouth or through the skin. Usually a form called *oestradiol* is used and the body is given the task of converting it to oestrone. So either oestrogen or progesterone can be used to help menopausal symptoms, but for most women who do not have PMS the preference is for oestrogen tablets, skin patches or implants.

One problem occurring after the menopause is osteoporosis, or brittle bone disease. This is likely to occur if a woman's mother has, or had, a 'dowager's hump' or fractures of the wrist or hip; in those who have previously taken steroids or had thyroid disease; those who in the past had anorexia, bulimia, loss of regular menstruation (other than during pregnancy) for more than six months; those committed athletes and ballet dancers who in their youth trained excessively and those who were sterilized before the age of 35 years. All these women are at risk and their chances of developing osteoporosis can be estimated by a bone mineral density scan. Professor J. Prior of Vancouver has shown how progesterone can be used to increase bone mineral density as successfully as oestrogen. If osteoporosis is already present, a special drug, *ethidronate* (Didronel) helps to build up the bones in addition to progesterone or oestrogen. Ethidronate is given for two weeks every three months.

Chapter 11

OTHER HORMONAL APPROACHES

This chapter deals with the hormonal treatments for PMS (other than progesterone, discussed in the previous chapter) which are likely to be given by medical professionals – gynaecologists and general practitioners. These include progestogens and the many uses to which they are put, and the hormones designed to eliminate ovulation (such as oral contraceptives, oestrogen, and man-made forms of gonadotrophin releasing hormone). They are all excellent treatments for other gynaecological problems as well, but in this chapter they are considered for treatment of PMS.

PROGESTOGENS

Progestogens, or *Progestins*, as the Americans tend to call them, have already been mentioned in Chapter 10. They are drugs which have been developed in laboratories and can all cause menstrual-type bleeding if the patient takes them, together with oestrogen, for a few days and then stops – any drug that does this is said to pass the 'Clauberg test' and is defined as a progestogen. They are alien to the human body. Some progestogens need a dose as little as 2,000 times lower than natural progesterone to cause vaginal bleeding. But, as we saw in Chapter 10, progestogens are different to progesterone in many other respects, and in some ways they even have the opposite actions to progesterone. In fact, very few medical or gynaecological books emphasize the differences between natural progesterone and the man-made progestogens; even the *British National Pharmacopoeia* does not distinguish them.

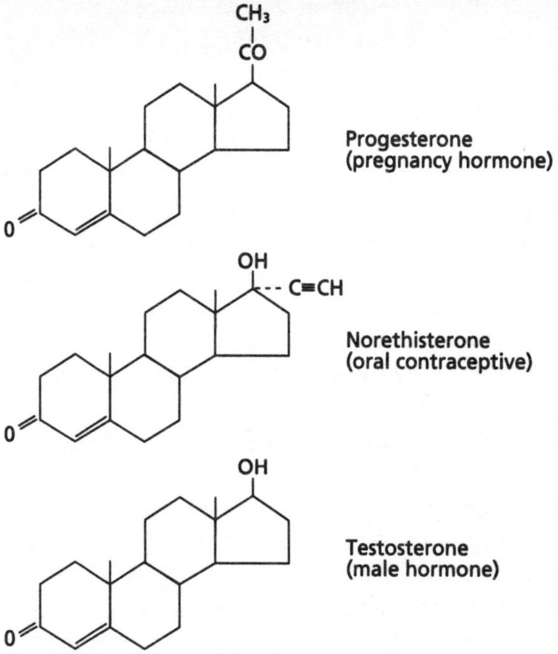

Figure 37: Formulae of progesterone, a progestogen and testosterone: which compound does norethisterone resemble?

The biochemists developed progestogens hoping to find a type of progesterone which would be effective if given by mouth or long-acting injection. The disadvantage of having to use progesterone by daily injections was recognized in the 1940s, and it was only in the 1960s that suppositories were developed. The main reason for finding such a drug was to make an oral contraceptive pill possible. It was known that oestrogen alone would work reasonably well as a contraceptive, and oestrogen, which does not even faintly resemble progesterone in its molecular structure, can be taken by mouth.

The trouble was, it was also known that oestrogen alone would build up the lining of the womb, as occurs naturally in the first half of the cycle, but would not cause bleeding. As we have seen, it is progesterone which does that job. Without menstrual bleeding, the risk of cancer was too great. Thus the great prize, the contraceptive pill – which has transformed the lives of millions of women, upturned the sexual ethics of half the world and (by the way) made billions for the manufacturers – was in sight if only a drug could be found which would produce withdrawal bleeding when stopped and which could be taken by mouth.

In the end, the biochemists were successful in their search, though the progestogens they developed have a lot in common with the male hormone, testosterone, which can also be taken by mouth. The common ones, *norethisterone* (Primulut N), *medroxyprogesterone acetate* (Provera), *dydrogesterone* (Duphaston), *norethyndrel, norgesterel* (Neogest), *norgestimate* (Celest) and *levonorgestrel* (Norgeston) can all be given by mouth; *medroxyprogesterone acetate* (Provera) can also be used as a long-acting injection, as can *hydroxyprogesterone hexanoate* (Prolutin Depot).

When a woman takes progesterone, the level of progesterone in the blood rises, of course, but when progestogens are given the blood progesterone level drops (see Chapter 5). As I said in the last chapter, a reasonable assumption is that the progestogen, which can 'fool' the body into having a period, can also fool the body into thinking there's more progesterone in the blood than there really is. Whatever the reason, a drop in progesterone blood level will make PMS worse.

Progesterone molecules in the blood pass into the cells and on to the nucleus of the cells by being attached to progesterone receptors which 'bind' on to them and transport them into the cell and on to the nucleus where (we think) they 'turn on' certain sequences of DNA. But progestogens won't bind properly to the progesterone receptors. Imagine that the progesterone receptor is a front door lock and progesterone is the key. A progestogen is close enough to fit into the lock, but not close enough to open it. The problem is that while the wrong key is in the lock, the right one can't get in. There's no one to pull the wrong one out.

In other ways it is clearer to think of the receptors as robot messengers who wait by the cell until a molecule of progesterone drifts by in the blood; they then grab it, dive through the cell wall with it and take it on to the nucleus where it's needed.

Progestogens are very useful drugs to the gynaecologists. They are used to reduce bleeding in those with very heavy periods, to help those who have irregular bleeding, and to ensure bleeding at the end of a month's course of oestrogen in HRT after the menopause. Most progestogens, but not dydrogesterone (Duphaston), are themselves contraceptives and all contraceptive pills contain progestogens, either with oestrogen, as in the combined pill, or alone as in the progestogen-only pill.

Progestogens Cause Fetal Malformation

Progesterone is the pregnancy hormone and is present in the body in massive amounts during pregnancy. Progestogens not only prevent pregnancies but, if used during pregnancy, they harm the developing baby, causing a female to have masculine features. This is not surprising when it is appreciated that many of the progestogens are developed from testosterone and have similar chemical formulae (see Figure 37).

Hormone Replacement Therapy (HRT)

We saw a moment ago that oestrogen must not be given to women continuously, as there is a danger that the lining of the womb will become too thickened and a risk of cancer may occur. Nature's way is to shed the lining of the womb every month and start a new one. Now, contraception is by no means the only reason for giving a woman oestrogen. HRT is the usual way of treating menopausal problems and *osteoporosis*, the thinning of the bones which occurs in so many women after the menopause and puts them at risk of dangerous fractures.

So, to ensure regular bleeding in HRT, every month's course of oestrogen includes some progestogen at the end to produce vaginal bleeding. When women have HRT they may find that at the end of each course they develop PMS-like symptoms produced by the progestogens in the HRT. These symptoms can be unpleasant and severe, and many opt instead for a hysterectomy, for without a uterus oestrogen can be given continuously to relieve menopausal symptoms – no lining = no build-up of lining = no cancer. There is always the alternative of using progesterone instead of progestogens to produce the necessary vaginal bleeding.

But, as we saw in Chapter 4, it now seems that progesterone

also works against osteoporosis. In every woman's bones, little pits are constantly forming and being filled up with new bone. It's Nature's way of keeping the bones strong. In postmenopausal women, the pits tend to form but not get filled up. Oestrogen seems to stop the pits from forming; progesterone causes them to be filled up. In the end, it seems, progesterone will turn out to be the better method for the bones, and it doesn't cause PMS-like symptoms in HRT.

Who's for Progestogens?

As long ago as 1959, a controlled trial of 'new' progestogens in the treatment of PMS was reported in the British Medical Journal by this author. Fifty-eight volunteers suffering from severe PMS, who all had complete relief from progesterone injections, were given oral progestogens. Of the 58 volunteers, 36 per cent benefited from ethisterone, 42 per cent from dimethisterone and 40 per cent from norethisterone, but within three months all the volunteers wanted to return to the progesterone injections, which they knew brought them full relief from their symptoms.

The progestogens do have their uses, though: if the patient's major problem is heavy menstruation, dysmenorrhoea, irregular menstruation or Mittelschmerz (midcycle pain), then progestogens may be the answer. For those having trouble with the progestogens at the end of the HRT course, we have just seen that it may be better to change to progesterone rather than have a hysterectomy.

ELIMINATING OVULATION

We know that PMS is a disease which starts and/or gets worse at times when (excluding pregnancy) for one reason or another there has been an absence of three or more months without menstruation. It is naïve to imagine that if we eliminate ovulation, PMS will also disappear. PMS is known to occur in cycles in which ovulation occurs as well as in anovular cycles in which ovulation does not occur. Nevertheless there are gynaecologists who believe in treating PMS by preventing ovulation, which can easily be achieved by five different methods.

> **Elimination of Ovulation**
> 1. Oral contraceptives
> 2. Continuous progestogens (discussed above)
> 3. Oestrogens
> 4. Danazol
> 5. GnRH agonists

Oral Contraceptives

Oral contraceptives have already been mentioned, also the fact that they are not helpful in PMS (see Chapter 5), although they do benefit those with heavy bleeding, irregular menstruation or spasmodic dysmenorrhoea. Some workers have studied the number of Pill-users who have PMS and how badly they get it, compared to non-users of the Pill. They found that PMS was less common and less severe in Pill-users, so now both lay people and doctors often think that the Pill is the answer. What the researchers did not consider in their studies is that among the non-users whom they used for comparison were a lot of PMS sufferers who had tried the Pill, found it unsatisfactory and stopped. Therefore a lot of the Pill-users in the studies were those who naturally didn't have PMS anyway – a lot of PMS sufferers had already been 'filtered out' into the non-Pill group.

Oestrogen

Oestrogen can be given by tablets, patches or implants. At the start PMS sufferers may benefit when on the oestrogen alone, but their problems start and increase when the progestogens are added. We have seen that oestrogens, for whatever reason they are given, thicken the endometrium (the lining of the womb), so if oestrogens are given it is always necessary to ensure that the lining is shed every month, and that this is usually achieved by giving progestogens each month, so that on stopping there will be vaginal bleeding. But as previously mentioned, the progestogens lower the blood progesterone level and make any PMS symptoms worse. Watson and Studd noted that as many as 10 per cent of women receiving oestrogen implants found the deterioration in PMS so severe when receiving regular oestrogen implants with cyclical progestogens that they opted for a hysterectomy. After a hysterectomy oestrogen can be given continuously without the need for progestogens.

Danazol

Danazol is an ultra-strong progestogen. It prevents ovulation by reducing oestrogen and by interfering with progesterone-receptor and androgen-receptor binding. It is useful in the treatment of endometriosis, causing the decay of the misplaced endometrial cells (see Chapter 2), and also in patients with bad dysmenorrhoea and breast tenderness, but it does not have much effect on the psychological symptoms of PMS. However, the side effects are the biggest problem; not many women want to risk weight gain, acne, masculinization (such as facial hair and deepening of the voice) as well as the long-term side effect of osteoporosis. If Danazol is used for PMS, low doses and regular frequent checkups are important.

GnRH Agonists and Antagonists

Gonadotrophin releasing hormone (better known as *GnRH*) is the chemical which comes from the menstrual controlling centre in the hypothalamus of the brain and stimulates the pituitary gland into producing the two hormones which act on the ovaries, the *follicle stimulating hormone (FSH)* and the *luteinizing hormone (LH)* (see Figure 18, page 46). Biochemists have now made drugs which act in the same way as GnRH, called *GnRH agonists*, and also drugs which stop the action of GnRH and are known as *GnRH antagonists*. They are very expensive and still in the experimental stage, so nothing is known of their long-term effects. Ovulation is suppressed, which means that most women develop hot flushes and vaginal dryness, while the pseudo-menopause which occurs increases the risk of heart disease and osteoporosis. At present, although GnRH agonists seem promising, their use is limited to six months, which is not very helpful with a long-term disease such as PMS.

Chapter 12

SURGICAL OPTIONS

It is important to remember that the major surgical operations usually performed to 'cure' PMS are permanent. There is no going back. It's not like stopping tablets, where after a time the body reverts to its previous state. This does not matter so much when contemplating a *D & C* or an *EUA*, but it is of vital importance when deciding whether to have a sterilization, hysterectomy and/or oophorectomy. (All these terms will be explained in a moment.) Even after a laparoscopy, when it has healed up there may be adhesions which can cause problems later. Hysterectomy, with or without oophorectomy, makes a woman infertile; this is a very important consideration for younger sufferers, although not of such importance for those approaching the menopause and who have completed their family. Nevertheless, even these older women should stop to consider the large number of people every year who want to have a sterilization reversed; a simple sterilization is sometimes reversible (though the increased PMS will continue), but a hysterectomy is absolutely final.

Perhaps it should also be mentioned that there is a very slight risk (about a one in a million chance) of dying from the anaesthetic. Because of this, before having any operation you will need to sign a consent form allowing the surgeon to take any steps considered necessary should an unexpected problem occur while you are under the anaesthetic.

D & C

This is the commonest of gynaecological operations; often the patient is in and out of hospital the same day. The mysterious letters stand for *Dilatation and Curettage*. 'Curettage' means scraping away a small amount of tissue from the womb. This is done by inserting a small instrument into the vagina, stretching or *dilating* the cervix (the opening to the womb) and then removing a bit of the lining, to be examined under a microscope to ensure there are no cancerous or abnormal cells. It is never done for the *treatment* of PMS, but may be done to make certain all is well and to exclude other problems before proceeding to treat the underlying PMS. If, for example, there has been heavy or irregular bleeding, perhaps from a polyp, then a D & C will spot the problem. After a D & C, young teenagers who suffered from spasmodic dysmenorrhoea may find that their symptoms vanish.

Nowadays D & Cs are not performed very frequently, as the inside of the womb can be inspected through a tiny periscope which can be inserted into the womb, and small sections of the lining can be removed for microscopical examination while the patient is conscious and on the gynaecologist's couch.

EUA

EUA is the gynaecological term for 'examination under anaesthetic'. This, too, is usually performed as a day case. When the patient is fully relaxed under an anaesthetic, it is easier to feel if there is any abnormal lump in the abdomen, for instance an ovarian cyst, a fibroid or an enlarged uterus. Also, if it is necessary to perform a vaginal examination on a very young girl with an intact hymen, it is often better for it to be done while she is in the deep sleep of an anaesthetic.

Again, this is not done for the relief of PMS, but to make sure that there is nothing else wrong. Today, a simple *ultrasonic pelvic scan* will detect an ovarian cyst, polycystic ovary, fibroid or an enlarged uterus, so EUAs are rarely performed these days. No anaesthetic is necessary for a scan, but the patient may be asked to fill up her bladder by drinking a lot of liquid one hour before, because with a full bladder the uterus and ovaries are lifted up and out of the pelvis into the abdomen and can be seen more easily.

LAPAROSCOPY AND LAPARECTOMY

In both these operations the contents of the abdomen are looked at, or *visualized*.

Laparoscopy is keyhole surgery in which two small incisions are made into the abdomen; a periscope is inserted through one of the holes and any instruments which might be needed go through the other. It is a minor operation, so the patient can normally leave hospital the next day.

In a laparectomy, the abdomen is opened up and thoroughly inspected, but it leaves a scar three to five inches in length, which will need to heal; this means several days in hospital.

These are the only ways in which endometriosis can be diagnosed, endometrial tissue can be removed and ovarian cysts can be *aspirated*, or emptied of fluid.

STERILIZATION

Among the vast number of PMS sufferers are many women who have completed their family and who find that the Pill does not suit them, or causes serious symptoms – including PMS. They often imagine that once they have a reliable method of contraception, such as sterilization, many of their other problems will disappear. Unfortunately, sterilization is likely to increase PMS, not cure it (see Chapter 1). Contrary to popular belief, it doesn't matter which way the sterilization is done, whether the Fallopian tubes are blocked by clamps, clips, sutures, cautery or cutting; it's all the same in the end (see Figure 5, page 14).

Exactly why there is this increase in severity of PMS after such a simple operation is a frequent topic of medical conversation. It may be because the ovarian nerve, artery and vein are closely attached to the Fallopian tube as it goes from the uterus to the ovary, and it has been shown that following sterilization there is a lower output of progesterone from the ovaries. Another school of thought tends to blame the many progesterone receptors within the Fallopian tubes. It is known that even if the tubes are subsequently rejoined or reopened again, and regardless of whether or not a pregnancy results, the PMS does not improve.

HYSTERECTOMY

Hysterectomy seems such a straightforward solution to the problem of PMS. Remove the offending organ, the womb, which creates such havoc each month during the build-up to menstruation, and all will be well. But that is wishful thinking, unfortunately; it is not as simple as that. About six to 12 months after the operation, the cyclical PMS symptoms will return, although of course without the womb there is no menstrual bleeding or pain.

Even some women who previously didn't have PMS at all find that after a hysterectomy they get PMS symptoms at approximately monthly intervals. When you look at the matter more closely, it's not really surprising. After all, taking away the uterus in the pelvis does not affect the menstrual controlling centre in the brain, nor the activity of the progesterone receptors present in most of the cells of the body. The menstrual clock is still ticking away there in the brain; there's no way it can 'know' that it might as well switch off because the womb has gone; and as long as it continues, the rest of the body will react in the usual cyclical way, even if the womb has been taken out.

The gynaecologist who does the hysterectomy does not see the end result of the operation two or three years later, and remains blissfully unaware that the patient is still suffering from cyclical symptoms. It is then left to the general practitioner to deal with the 'problem patient'. At first the long-suffering patient will probably be offered HRT, but when that is unsuccessful she is likely to be referred to the psychiatrist, neurologist, rheumatologist, etc., etc.

There are many good reasons for having a hysterectomy, but PMS is not one of them. Cancer, endometriosis and large fibroids are well-recognized problems which can be treated by hysterectomy. Heavy menstrual bleeding, particularly if it is causing anaemia, used to be another reason, but nowadays many cases of *menorrhagia*, as heavy menstruation is called, can be helped by *endometrial resection*. This is a simple operation in which only a part of the lining of the womb is eliminated by a laser beam, so that at future menstruations there is a smaller lining to come away and bleeding is considerably lessened.

After a hysterectomy the ovaries may weaken, so that there is

	Jan	Feb	Mar	Apr	May	Jun	Jul
1					X		
2					X		
3				X	X		
4				X			
5				X			
6				X			
7			X	X			
8			X				
9		X	X				
10		X					
11		X					
12		X					
13	X	X					
14	X						
15	X						
16	X						
17							
18							
19							X
20							X
21						X	X
22						X	
23						X	
24						X	
25							
26					X		
27					X		
28					X		
29							
30				X			
31							

Figure 38: Menstrual chart one year after a hysterectomy
(X = symptoms)

an oestrogen deficiency which causes menopausal symptoms in addition to PMS. This can be corrected by oestrogen treatment, which can be given continuously as there is now no longer any risk of causing too thick a lining with the possibility of nasty side effects (see Chapter 11). Progesterone can always be given continuously at the same time as oestrogen.

Those who are still suffering cyclical PMS symptoms after a hysterectomy are advised to keep their usual menstrual chart. The cyclic pattern of any symptoms will still show up, even if there is no more menstruation to mark on the chart (Figure 38).

PMS can still be successfully treated with the three-hourly starch diet (Chapter 6) and progesterone (Chapter 10), although after a hysterectomy progesterone needs to be given continuously and not in bi-weekly courses.

OOPHORECTOMY

Oophorectomy is the removal of one or both ovaries. It is often done together with a hysterectomy. The removal of one ovary often makes little or no difference to fertility, and regular ovulatory menstruation may continue, nor does it always cause or increase the severity of PMS. However, after the removal of both ovaries there will be acute menopausal symptoms, which require continuous oestrogen treatment given by tablets, patches, or implant. PMS is not necessarily eliminated. If there is a lessening or complete absence of sex drive after the operation, a small testosterone pellet may be implanted together with the oestrogen implant. Continuous progesterone can be given together with oestrogen therapy if PMS comes back after a few months.

The upheaval in the menstrual controlling centre caused by a bilateral (double) oophorectomy with hysterectomy often dulls the PMS symptoms for six to twelve months before they return – another reason why hospital doctors and others who do not have to cope with the long-term effects believe that this operation cures PMS.

Careful thought needs to be given before deciding on a bilateral oophorectomy. The usual test is to see if the PMS will disappear on Danazol treatment or with GnRH agonists (see Chapter 11), as these drugs produce a 'medical oophorectomy' – the ovaries, though still present, stop working, just as if they had been taken out. If one of these treatments proves successful after six or more months, then it suggests that bilateral oophorectomy and hysterectomy may be the answer in cases of severe PMS occurring in a woman who is nearing the menopause. A hysterectomy will be needed at the same time, as otherwise it will still be necessary to produce regular bleeding of the lining of the womb with oestrogen treatment, in order to prevent problems there.

Chapter 13

PROGESTERONE AND CONCEPTION, PREGNANCY AND CONTRACEPTION

It is a well-recognized fact about PMS that most sufferers are free of their monthly problems when pregnant, or at least during the second half of pregnancy. This is because the placenta produces huge amounts of progesterone to keep the pregnancy going – it may raise the level of progesterone in the blood to 40 or even 50 times the greatest amount found in non-pregnant women. However, there are a few women who continue to experience their PMS symptoms daily during later pregnancy, and these women are the ones who are most at risk of developing *pre-eclampsia* (page 150).

CONCEPTION

Women who suffer from PMS usually have no difficulty in conceiving. When patients who are receiving progesterone therapy are ready to become pregnant, they are advised to start their usual course of progesterone two to four days later and continue until the pregnancy is confirmed. Then they should phone for further advice. They will be asked if they have any of the usual pregnancy problems – nausea, vomiting, headaches, excessive tiredness or depression. These are common symptoms in early pregnancy and can be relieved by increasing their current dose of progesterone.

If a woman is not experiencing any of these pregnancy symptoms, she can reduce her usual dose of progesterone slowly, week by week. On the other hand if these pregnancy symptoms are present, the patient should increase her dose of progesterone every few days until she feels really well. She will usually be asked to report her progress on the phone, week by week until the symptoms are stabilized. Often progesterone may be needed until the placenta is fully functioning and producing large amounts, which is generally about the fourth month. (See Figure 40 on page 154, which indicates the beneficial effects of progesterone on the children of mothers given progesterone in early pregnancy.)

Recent advances in the use of ultrasound pelvic scans have revealed just how often conception occurs only to be followed by failure of the fertilized ovum to embed itself into the lining of the womb, even in perfectly normal, fertile women. This results in an early miscarriage even before the woman has considered the possibility of a pregnancy, or it may even happen as early as the time of the next expected period. The only telltale sign may be unexpectedly heavy menstrual bleeding and/or more pain than usual.

Defective Luteal Phase

Progesterone is the pregnancy hormone. If there is too short an interval between ovulation and menstruation, this is known as a *defective luteal phase*. The short interval, of less than 12 days, means that there has not been a high enough progesterone level and this may result in an early miscarriage, due to failure of the fertilized egg to embed itself in the lining of the womb. This hazard can be overcome by ensuring there is sufficient progesterone after ovulation and until the placenta has started producing enough on its own. It means continuing progesterone therapy until about the fourth month of pregnancy.

In Vitro Fertilization

Those unfortunate women who, for one reason or another, have difficulty in conceiving naturally and need *in vitro* fertilization (IVF) will also require progesterone from the time of implantation until the placenta is producing enough progesterone to keep the embryo going. There are several different types of IVF treatment, but they will all need plenty of progesterone in the first few weeks.

PREGNANCY

Morning Sickness

Morning sickness in early pregnancy is another hazard for PMS sufferers. In fact, many will tell you that the name is wrong – they are sick all day, not just in the morning. When this problem is severe it is called *hyperemesis* (from the Greek words *hyper*, meaning 'excessive' and *emesis*, meaning 'vomiting'). This seems to mean that in former times doctors (who were always male, of course) considered mild vomiting in early pregnancy to be quite natural, something to be expected and which the women should learn to accept. It's a pity they never had to go through it! In fact it is caused by a hormonal imbalance before the placenta is fully formed, and usually improves by about the 16th week of pregnancy. Using progesterone will help this problem, too.

Habitual Miscarriages

When a woman has had several miscarriages, she is naturally anxious that everything medically possible is done to ensure that she has a normal full-term pregnancy – and, not surprisingly, she will often be given progesterone therapy to ensure this. There are many causes of miscarriages, including chromosomal defects, about which little can be done at present, but they may be due to anatomical abnormalities such as a lax cervix (opening to the womb), which can be stitched up until labour starts. There are also women who suffer from excessive vomiting and pregnancy symptoms immediately they become pregnant, and these are the ones most likely to benefit from progesterone given in a dose high enough to remove their symptoms. Among many patients thus treated over the years, the author has treated two women who had both had nine previous miscarriages and who were both given progesterone therapy; both were later delivered successfully of healthy babies at the City of London Maternity Hospital.

Threatened Miscarriages

Bleeding in early pregnancy is always a worry; the patient is naturally wondering whether it is the end of the pregnancy or not. If the bleeding is scanty and does not contain clots or fetal tissue, then with rest there is a chance that all will be well and that a normal pregnancy will continue. This applies particularly if the bleeding comes at the expected time of the first missed period. If it is accompanied by excessive vomiting and early pregnancy symptoms, then again the patient will benefit from progesterone therapy in a dose sufficient to ease the symptoms. However, after the delivery the doctor is left wondering if the pregnancy would have continued even if progesterone had not been given.

Pre-eclampsia

Pre-eclampsia was previously known as 'toxaemia of pregnancy' and is often referred to as *PET*, or *pre-eclamptic toxaemia*. The word *toxaemia* means 'blood-poisoning'; *pre* means 'before', and the *eclampsia* refers to the convulsions which can sometimes occur in severe cases of PET, often resulting in the death of the mother or the baby. It is still one of the commonest causes of both infant and maternal deaths in Britain and throughout the world.

We still don't know exactly what causes PET, although all over the world scientists are searching for a better understanding of the disease process. It is known that harmful changes occur in the endothelial cells (the cells lining the inside of blood vessels) of the womb and placenta, where plaques begin to form between the 16th and 20th week of pregnancy, but the disease does not show until late pregnancy when there is a rise in blood pressure, excessive weight gain, swelling of the ankles and protein in the urine.

In the first-ever description of 'Premenstrual Syndrome', in the *British Medical Journal* in 1953 by Dr Raymond Greene and this author, it was noted that twice as many PMS sufferers had been hospitalized because of pre-eclampsia in a previous pregnancy compared with the normal number of cases of pre-eclampsia in the general population. This led to a survey of 825 women, published in the *British Medical Journal* in 1955, which confirmed that the 192 women who had previously suffered from pre-eclampsia had a 86 per cent incidence of PMS compared with 27 per cent among those whose pregnancy had been normal (Figure

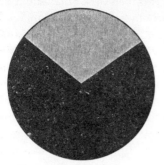 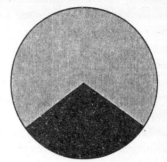

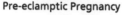

Pre-eclamptic Pregnancy   Normal Controls

Figure 39: Incidence of PMS after a normal pregnancy (right) and one complicated by pre-eclampsia (left)

39). This suggested a link between pre-eclampsia and PMS.

The women in the survey were interviewed personally by the author, who noted that the symptoms experienced by those who had pre-eclampsia during middle and late pregnancy were the same as those which they subsequently experienced during their PMS. For instance, the biggest problem for some women was headaches throughout pregnancy, and these women were later troubled by premenstrual headaches; others were worried by depression or backache, in each case it was these same symptoms which later caused problems before their periods.

In the 1950s, a few women with severe PMS including premenstrual epilepsy, asthma and migraine, were tested daily for weight, blood pressure and protein in their urine, the same tests as are done during antenatal examinations in order to spot PET. These examinations showed that women with severe PMS also had an increase in weight, blood pressure and developed protein in their urine before menstruation, but these measurements were normal after menstruation. These patients were then treated with daily progesterone injections and the daily examinations continued, but with progesterone there was no weight gain, no rise in blood pressure and no protein in the urine. They were free from symptoms.

In another survey by this author, published in the *Lancet* in 1960, 640 women attending the antenatal clinic of University College Hospital, London, were asked between the 16th and 28th weeks of their pregnancy whether they felt as well as they did before they became pregnant. Their names and hospital number were then entered either into a book marked 'YES' or one marked 'NO'. The patients' records were later studied and it was found that among those women who felt ill during the middle months of pregnancy, 25 per cent developed pre-eclampsia compared with only 10 per cent among those who felt well. The complaints of the women who were not feeling well in the middle months of pregnancy, and who later developed pre-eclampsia, are shown here:

Symptoms in the middle months of pregnancy in those who later developed pre-eclampsia

Lethargy	88 per cent	Backache	44 per cent
Nausea and		Headache	35 per cent
vomiting	65 per cent	Vertigo	26 per cent
Depression	52 per cent	Fainting	12 per cent

These facts all suggested that there was a marked similarity between pre-eclampsia and PMS – in fact, in the days when pre-eclampsia was called 'toxaemia of pregnancy', it was suggested that PMS should be called 'toxaemia of menstruation'. Both have an early first stage of symptoms, followed in severe cases by the

---

Similarity of PMS and pre-eclampsia

First stage:
- Nausea and vomiting
- Lethargy
- Depression
- Headache
- Irritability
- Backache
- Fainting

Second Stage:
- Weight gain
- Swelling of ankles and fingers
- Rise of blood pressure
- Protein in the urine

Third Stage
- Epileptic fits, preceded by severe headache
- Eclamptic convulsions, preceded by severe headache

---

second stage of weight gain, rise in blood pressure and protein in the urine, and if the disease progresses even further there is a third stage of fits, either eclamptic convulsions or epileptic fits.

Because progesterone is successful in PMS if used early, it was decided to use progesterone in controlled trials for pre-eclampsia, first by injection (1962) and later by suppository (1972).

Volunteers attending the antenatal clinic of Chase Farm Hospital, Enfield, who were in the middle months of pregnancy and complaining of pregnancy symptoms, were allocated randomly to receive either progesterone or treatment which would relieve their symptoms until they were well again or until their baby was born. It proved easy enough to relieve symptoms in both groups of 296 pregnant women, but in the group of those receiving progesterone only 3 per cent developed pre-eclampsia, compared with the symptomatic treatment groups in which 11 per cent developed pre-eclampsia.

Progesterone treatment for pre-eclampsia has proved effective in Egypt and Japan, but in Britain doctors have feared that progesterone in pregnancy would have the same harmful effects on the fetus as the artificial man-made progestogens. Also, in Britain consultant obstetricians do not usually see antenatal patients until the late stage of pregnancy, when they would much prefer to have proof of tests showing abnormal blood pressure and protein in the urine, rather than rely on a woman's account of how she feels.

Antenatal Progesterone and the Fetus

In the late 1950s pregnant women suffering from morning sickness were successfully treated with progesterone injections. Several of these children were in the author's general practice. One morning a patient asked me if I had attended the local school's prize-giving the previous day. When I asked 'Why?' I was told that I had delivered many of the prizewinners. This roused my curiosity, and at coffee break the files of the named prizewinners were fetched out and looked at. I noticed with surprise that the prizewinners' mothers had received progesterone for morning sickness during their pregnancies.

The local Director of Education was most interested and asked for a list of 40 local children, including the six prizewinners and others who had received progesterone in the womb. He hecked with the headmasters if the other 'progesterone children' were also bright. Indeed, a lot of the children who received progesterone in the womb appeared to be brighter than average.

There then followed a full-scale survey of the children of all mothers who had received progesterone at the City of London Maternity Hospital between 1959 and 1961. The children were then 9–10 years old and scattered around London and various parts of Britain, and they were each matched with a 'control' – the next baby in the labour ward register. The babies' progress could then be compared with these controls. The school heads were asked to grade each child as average, below average or above average in English, arithmetic, verbal reasoning, craftwork and physical education (Figure 40).

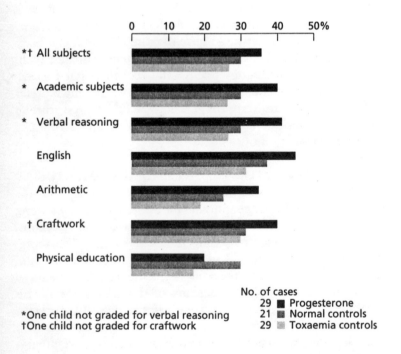

Figure 40: Above-average grades of 79 children 9–10 years old (from K. Dalton , British Journal of Psychiatry 516: 114, 1377, 1968)

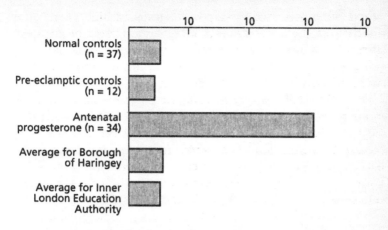

Figure 41: University places gained by 'progesterone children' and controls

Further results confirmed that among the 'progesterone children', the best results were among those who received high doses compared with low doses, long courses compared with short courses and before the 16th week of pregnancy compared with later in pregnancy. This was true in all the academic subjects: English, arithmetic and verbal reasoning but not in physical education or craftwork. In medical terms, the results showed that the effect of progesterone on intelligence was 'dose related' – the more the better.

The children were followed up until the age of 20 years, when they showed better exam (O and A level) results than did the controls. Finally, 32 per cent of the 'progesterone children' went on to university, compared with only 6 per cent of the controls, and 6 per cent is also the average number for the borough of Haringey and the Inner London Education Authority who entered university during those years (Figure 41). Although the survey has now finished I can record anecdotally that the 'progesterone children' have married and have had no problems with fertility.

In 1960 the first reports appeared of abnormalities to a fetus exposed to progestogens – it was found that they caused masculinization of female babies. At that time, the differences between progestogens and progesterone were not well understood, so progesterone was no longer used for the relief of morning sickness in pregnancy. In retrospect, it is not surprising that these abnormalities occurred, as the progestogens then used were all related to the male hormone testosterone. However, with the arrival of *in vitro* fertilization ('test-tube babies') it has been recognized that progesterone is an essential hormone of pregnancy, and it has been given to women when the fertilized egg is planted in the womb and until the placenta is producing adequate progesterone. So, in the future we can hope to see more of these intelligent 'progesterone children'.

Postnatal Depression

Postnatal depression (PND) is really the wrong name for an illness which affects 10 per cent of new mothers after their baby's birth, because depression is rarely the first symptom to appear and in many cases there is never any depression at all. Women who have suffered from PND can give much better descriptions of how they felt at the beginning of their illness, describing the sleeplessness and feeling 'not with it' – 'distant' – 'shattered' – 'confused' – 'losing touch' – 'muddled' – 'out of control' – 'high, gloriously high' – 'mind going round' – 'couldn't talk/wouldn't go out/kept the curtains drawn each day' – 'spent money like there was no tomorrow' – 'angry' and 'panicky'.

It can be a horrifying experience for a partner to come face-to-face with the changed personality of the new mother who was previously calm and is now so anxious, previously alert and active but now dull and speechless, previously a successful career woman and now frightened to be left alone, previously carefree and now obsessional. As mentioned previously, postnatal depression, and its more severe cousin puerperal psychosis, are hormonal diseases which have a lot in common with PMS and frequently turn into PMS as time passes. As a PND sufferer gradually improves, she will find that her symptoms get better after menstruation, only to get worse again before the next menstruation, and with further progress she gradually reaches the stage when there is absence of symptoms after menstruation but many of the symptoms premenstrually. At this point the illness has changed to PMS.

Postnatal depression tends to occur in women who have

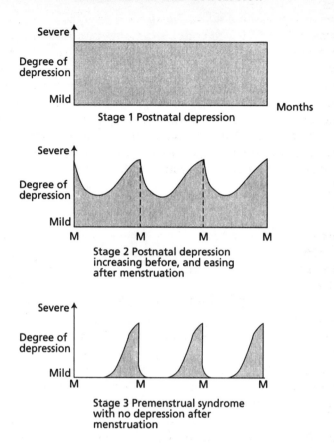

Figure 42: Stages of postnatal depression as it gradually changes to PMS (M = menstruation)

suffered from severe PMS and in those who have already suffered from postnatal depression or puerperal psychosis after a previous pregnancy, and it may come unexpectedly after a perfectly normal pregnancy and delivery. It can be successfully avoided if arrangements are made during the pregnancy with the general practitioner, obstetrician and midwife. After the baby has been safely delivered, the mother should be given the first of seven daily progesterone injections: of 100 mg followed by 400 mg progesterone suppositories twice daily for the next two months or until normal menstruation returns.

Progesterone for Postnatal Depression

Immediately after delivery, progesterone injections 100 mg daily for seven days, followed by progesterone suppositories 400 mg twice daily until the return of menstruation or for two months.

Menstruation is not likely to return until after breastfeeding has finished, so if the mother is feeling well and plans to continue breastfeeding for many months, the progesterone can be stopped after two months – but, if the symptoms come back, the progesterone should be restarted. When progesterone was first isolated in 1934, researchers thought that its job in the body was to prepare the breasts for breastfeeding. Progesterone helps breastfeeding and mothers need not worry that it will upset their babies.

Good News

When PMS sufferers have had adequate progesterone during pregnancy so that there have been no symptoms of pregnancy, no hyperemesis or rise of blood pressure, and if progesterone has been given after the delivery to prevent any postnatal depression, then there is about a 50/50 chance that the PMS will not return.

CONTRACEPTION

Contraception is often a problem for women with PMS. All contraceptive pills contain progestogens, and as has already been explained in Chapter 5, the artificial man-made progestogens lower the blood progesterone level and so increase the severity of PMS. This means that the Pill should be avoided. Again, it is known that PMS increases in severity after sterilization (see Chapter 1), so this rules out another popular method of contraception. The intra-uterine device, or *IUD*, is best not used by any woman who has had problems with pelvic infections or by young girls who have not been pregnant. Withdrawal as a method of contraception is very unreliable (and bad for the nerves!). So, apart from progesterone contraception, this leaves condoms – male or female – the diaphragm (or 'Dutch Cap') and vasectomy.

Nowadays a doctor would advise any woman with a new partner to use a condom for the first six months, until any risk of HIV or AIDS has passed.

Progesterone Contraception

Progesterone is as safe a contraceptive as the intra-uterine device or the progestogen-only pill, if used as follows: Start on Day 8 of the cycle with a low dose of progesterone, and keep it up until menstruation or – for PMS sufferers – the day when you start on the bigger, anti-PMS dose. A daily dose of 100 mg (half a 200 mg suppository) or a 400 mg suppository are equally effective. (Many women who will use 400 mg of progesterone two to six times daily from ovulation onwards prefer to take one 400 mg suppository in the follicular phase rather than having to get 200 mg suppositories as well.)

Progesterone contraception for PMS
- A low dose (100–200 mg) of progesterone from Day 8 of the cycle
- Increase to optimum progesterone dosage at ovulation
- Continue progesterone until menstruation.

A study of progesterone contraception in women with severe PMS showed 15 failures in 253 women who had used proges-terone contraception for an average of 5.82 years. This means a failure rate of 2.66 per 100 women/years (women/years is a ratio that encompasses 100 women using a method of contra-ception for one year, 50 women using it for two, etc.), which compares favourably with the recognized failure rate of the condom of 14, diaphragm of 12, rhythm method 24, and intra-uterine device of 2.5 per 100 women/years.

However, some women find that by starting progesterone early they start bleeding at, or shortly after, ovulation. They should be advised to lower the dose of daily progesterone from Day 8 to 100 mg daily and start their usual higher dose of progesterone about two days after ovulation. If extra bleeding still occurs, then it is best to use a condom or diaphragm until the normal time of starting their course of progesterone. Should attacks of diarrhoea occur when using progesterone, then contraception cannot be guaranteed and alternative methods are advised.

Chapter 14

THE SUCCESS RATES OF DIFFERENT PMS TREATMENTS

Perhaps it is not surprising that there are so many options for the treatment of a disease like PMS, which has at least 150 different symptoms and occurs across a wide age range in millions of women of all races, who are nevertheless all different individuals. Until there are greater scientific advances enabling us to understand more of the underlying biochemical problems at cellular level, we are all left to tread carefully through this minefield of treatment options. The key to success is the *holistic* approach – to treat each woman as an individual, rather than to lay down the law about one type of treatment to cure everybody.

It is interesting to see the changes in the popularity of various PMS treatments which have occurred during the last decade. In 1983, records of each patient's previous medication were noted when my analysis was carried out for the American Food and Drug Administration, who were investigating the use of progesterone. In 1993, a similar analysis was performed on all new patients attending the same (my) PMS Clinic in London, where

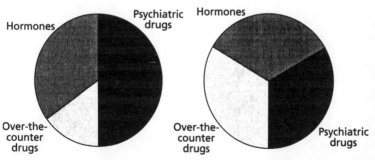

Figure 43: Treatments before attendance at the PMS Clinic 1983 (left) and 1993 (right)

patients are only seen on the recommendation of a doctor (Figure 43). In short, all patients had tried at least one kind of treatment before attending the Clinic, and because it was ineffective they sought further help, or what doctors call a 'second opinion'.

There was an interesting shift over the 10 years, with more women trying over-the-counter medication and fewer being given tranquillizing drugs by their general practitioner or psychiatrist (see Table 5).

Table 5: Medication Tried Before Attendance at a PMS Clinic in 1983 and 1993		
	1983	**1993**
Number interviewed	1096	81
	per cent	*per cent*
Tranquillizers	27	15
Antidepressants	23	30
Progestogens	20	30
Diuretics	11	4
Pyridoxine (B$_6$)	11	47
Progesterone	9	25
Contraceptive Pill	6	19
Analgesics	5	7
Oestrogen	4	9
HRT	3	7
Non-steroidal Anti-inflammatories	2	7
Bromocriptine	1	1

It has been pointed out that a lie, however big, will be accepted as the truth if it is repeated loudly enough and often enough. This seems to be the basis for the marked increase in the number of women who tried pyridoxine (vitamin B$_6$) and when it failed asked their doctors to refer them to the PMS Clinic. It was in 1983 that Schaumberg first alerted us to the dangers of Vitamin B$_6$ in producing deterioration of nerve endings (see Chapter 8). Yet the increase in the last decade of those who have tried pyridoxine reflects the success of the manufacturers' manipulation of non-medical journalists and agony aunts into writing repeatedly about the apparent effectiveness of B$_6$.

It is disappointing to see how often progestogens and the oral contraceptive pill were prescribed as a remedy for PMS. This reflects the ignorance of too many doctors in not appreciating the difference between natural progesterone and the man-made progestogens (see Chapter 10). This was brought home recently when the charity PMS Help offered a £2,000 prize to the doctor who could write the best essay of not more than 5,000 words on 'The differences between progesterone and the other progestogens'. The doctors who wanted to enter the competition and who therefore looked for information realized that it is a subject not covered by medical, gynaecological or pharma-cological textbooks – it required researching in medical journals. So who is to blame for their ignorance?

Progesterone use has increased during the last decade. The patients referred for a further opinion came because their doctors were unfamiliar with the rules of using progesterone suppositories (see Chapter 10). There is a need to teach doctors to help patients maintain a steady blood sugar level, to use a higher dose, to treat thrush effectively and to tailor individually the course to each woman's own menstrual cycle. Much of this work does not need to be done by the GPs themselves; it can be undertaken by the practice nurse, especially in helping women to keep their menstrual charts and supervising each individual's diet.

The fact that so much attention is being paid to the menopause at this time is reflected in the greater emphasis on the need to eliminate unpleasant menopausal symptoms and the dangers of osteoporosis. This is responsible for the increased use of oestrogen and HRT for PMS. Today, women in their early forties, and unfortunately also their doctors, too easily tend to blame all symptoms on the menopause, the average age of which is now nearer to 52 years. It is a bit like blaming all problems in a five-year-old on the approach of puberty, which will hit her in eight or 10 years' time.

It is satisfying to see the reduction in the use of diuretics (or water tablets). Gradually, doctors are realizing that diuretics are addictive and that they are not the answer to bloatedness or weight gain.

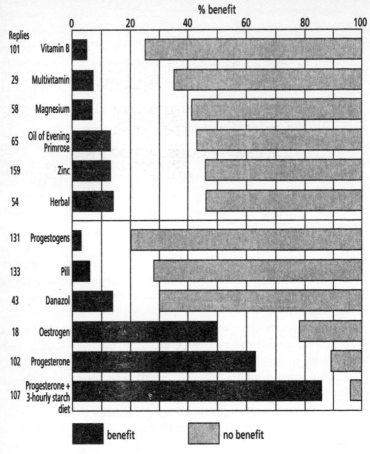

Figure 44: Benefit of over-the-counter medication for PMS

SURVEY OF PMS PATIENTS

In 1989, a survey of members of The National Association for Premenstrual Syndrome (NAPS) asked them to list the benefit or otherwise that they had received from various treatments. Questionnaires were returned by lay members (Figure 44), and the first 250 replies were analysed. We do not know how many of these women were diagnosed by doctors, and how many by themselves, but the chances are that they were relatively severe cases, as the average number of symptoms reported was 6.5.

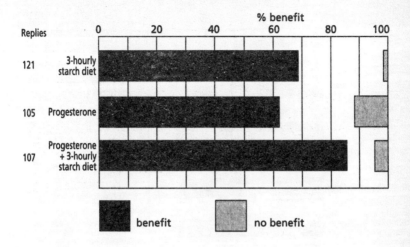

Figure 45: Benefit of hormone therapy plus the three-hourly starch diet for PMS

Some of the treatments were not reported in enough cases to be statistically significant, including hysterectomy (3 cases) and sterilization (32 cases – all failures).

I should mention that at that time NAPS was an excellent organization which had worked hard to promote the idea of eating starchy foods at three-hourly intervals, although they have since advocated a high-fibre carbohydrate diet, with much less success.

It is astonishing to note the complete failure of the vitamins and minerals which can be obtained over the counter. When a doctor writes a prescription, he or she certainly hopes for a better result than 7 to 13 per cent successful relief of symptoms. On the other hand, nowadays when the costs of a doctor's prescriptions are so carefully scrutinized, there may be a temptation to suggest vitamin B_6 on the grounds that it will save on the drug bill. However, Figure 45 demonstrates the beneficial effect of maintaining the three-hourly starch diet, which costs the NHS – and the patient – nothing! Even easier for the doctor, the patient can be taught about the diet and supervised by the practice nurse.

The failure of progestogens, oral contraceptives and Danazol

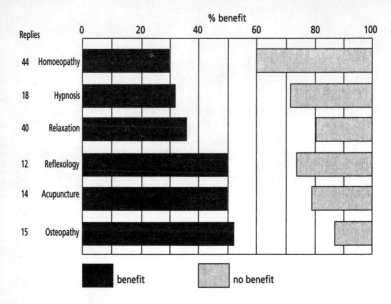

Figure 46: Benefit of alternative medicine for PMS

(see Figure 44) to bring relief is shattering. These treatments would all have been prescribed by registered medical practitioners, but were probably not followed up long enough to assess their value in relieving PMS. The beneficial effect of the three-hourly starch diet is very clearly shown.

The failure of progestogens to benefit PMS is in marked contrast to the relief obtained from progesterone, especially when combined with the three-hourly starch diet (Figure 45), which brought benefit to 86 per cent. Only 4 per cent received no relief at all from their symptoms.

The Alternative Practitioner

Compared with over-the-counter medications, a visit to an 'alternative' practitioner may seem to offer more hope (Figure 46). Is this because these practitioners tend to take a holistic view and because the consultation lasts longer? The harassed GP has only three to five minutes per consultation. On the other hand, the GP does have the advantage of knowing about the patient's previous illnesses and problems.

CLINICAL TRIALS

Medical scientists like to measure the effectiveness of treatment by doing a *clinical trial*. This is a planned experiment on a sample of patients, all with the same disease, giving half one type of treatment and the others another treatment. The effect of the different treatments are then compared in the two groups.

Problems with Trials

Many doctors refuse to try progesterone treatment because the clinical trials have not shown it to be effective. But there are a lot of problems with doing clinical trials for PMS. So far, no trials have been done using a high enough dose of progesterone, and none has studied the effect of progesterone together with a diet to prevent a drop in blood sugar level.

In a trial, patients are allotted at random to the treatment groups; they may not choose. This is the first hurdle with PMS clinical trials. It is well-nigh impossible to get a sample of PMS women all with the same type, timing, severity and mixture of PMS symptoms.

How Do You Judge a Treatment?

Ideally one compares the new drug with an old drug which is already recognized as the best treatment for that particular disease. A new drug to control high blood pressure or raised cholesterol level will be compared with the best old drug for treating these conditions, for example. Or one might compare a new pain-relieving drug with paracetamol in easing any pain after a minor operation, such as a laparoscopy, and note when and how often patients in either group ask for pain relief. This is not considered such a good trial, however, as it relies on the patient's pain tolerance, which we know varies between individuals, and it does not rely on precise measurements by an outside observer, such as can be obtained from a blood test or measure of blood pressure. A trial based on patients' opinions means that larger numbers of volunteers will be required to iron out the individual differences.

Now there are many conditions, like PMS, for which there is

no existing accepted treatment to compare with. How do you do a trial in such cases? Well, the obvious answer is to compare some patients who are getting the new treatment with other patients who are not being treated at all. There are at least two problems with this, though: one is that the patients know whether they are getting the treatment or not, and that this knowledge may affect the result. Especially in something like PMS, which is hard to measure, the fact that you know you are being treated may make you feel better. Therefore a *placebo* is used.

A placebo is basically a dummy pill made of something which is known to have no effect on the condition being tested. In a trial, those taking the placebo are not actually receiving any treatment at all, but they don't know whether they are getting the drug or a placebo so 'imaginary' effects should be ruled out.

In a *double-blind* trial, the doctors measuring the results don't know who is taking the placebo, either – only another worker, acting as a sort of referee, knows this until the measurements have been made and the results of the trial are ready to be worked out. This should rule out any cheating, deliberate or not, by the patients or the doctors. It has been found that a lot of patients involved in trials for all sorts of remedies actually get better on the placebo, at least for a while, because they *believe* that the remedy is doing them good.

The ultimate trial is a *double-blind crossover* trial, in which the placebo group and the group taking the medication are swapped over halfway through – again, the testers do not know who is in which group until the end of the trial.

This points up another problem with doing clinical trials. If you are treating patients who are quite ill, you know that the ones getting the placebo are not getting any help. Is it morally right to deny help to some patients just to obtain scientific data? After all, the doctors may be almost certain – or even 100 per cent certain – that the treatment works. In many instances they can see that without a placebo study. In the case of drugs for serious illnesses, it may become obvious before the end of the trial that the treatment is working; it then becomes unfair for the placebo group not to be getting the treatment, so the trial is stopped.

In the case of injections, the placebo – basically just water – would still have to be injected into the volunteers, which would be open to ethical objections on the grounds that it would be an invasion of the body. This is another reason why there have been no clinical trials to judge the effectiveness of progesterone injections in PMS. Nevertheless, a double-blind placebo-controlled trial remains the 'gold standard' of clinical trials.

Obviously, patients cannot be used in a trial without their consent; they must be volunteers. Volunteers must be willing to accept that they may very well have to go for four or six months without effective treatment, and those whose suffering is serious do not want to wait that long. They demand treatment immediately. This means that volunteers for PMS trials tend to be those with only mild or very moderate PMS, ones who can probably be relieved by diet alone.

Everybody knows that the way to treat diabetes is to give insulin, yet for this reason insulin treatment in diabetes has never been subjected to double-blind placebo-controlled trials. We *know* it works, and placebo trials would be immoral. There are plenty of other standard treatments which have never undergone a placebo trial because of this. Nevertheless, the same doctors who refuse to prescribe progesterone do not hesitate to prescribe insulin.

More Problems with PMS Trials

Exactly which patients are to be included in PMS trials, and how to find them, is another problem. In the US they will often put advertisements for volunteers in the newspapers, but there the volunteers are also likely to be paid and also provided with medication which they otherwise could not afford.

The definition of PMS is: 'The presence of symptoms before menstruation with complete absence of symptoms after menstruation,' but this is not precise enough for well-designed clinical trials. It must limit the days of symptoms strictly to no more than the 14 premenstrual days and insist that there must be a minimum of seven days after menstruation with no symptoms. In 1988 Dr Gwyneth Sampson and colleagues in Sheffield reported findings in their paper in the *British Journal of Psychiatry*, 'PMS, a double blind crossover study of treatment with dydrogesterone and placebo', but they included patients with just a *lessening* of symptoms after menstruation, rather than a complete absence; in short, it was a trial testing the efficacy of dydrogesterone (Duphaston) in *menstrual distress* (see Chapter 2), and not purely PMS. The study should have been better designed. By the way, the dydrogesterone eased pain at menstruation but increased breast tenderness.

Many controlled trials of PMS treatments allow symptoms *after menstruation* as well as before. Again, this is mixing up PMS sufferers and women with menstrual distress, which is bound to confuse the issue. The patient should have no other complicating disease, but Olsen in 1981 was in favour of studying PMS in women awaiting hysterectomy for anaemia and heavy bleeding, so they all had another complicating disease – anaemia.

PMS is a hormonal disease, and among the characteristics of hormonal diseases are the presence of both psychological and physical symptoms, so they are difficult to diagnose using a questionnaire. A good example of this is diabetes. Not many doctors would give a patient insulin merely on the result of a questionnaire which reported that she was often hungry, tired, thirsty, losing weight and passing water frequently, yet all these things are recognized by all doctors as symptoms of diabetes.

A questionnaire often used in PMS work is the *Moos Menstrual Distress Questionnaire*, designed by Professor Moos in 1968 to find out how much distress resulted from menstruation in different samples of women. It was not designed to be used to detect PMS alone, but all problems associated with menstruation, such as dysmenorrhoea. It consists of 47 questions which are answered on a six-point scale.

Recently, an American professor and his wife visited me and spoke about their new PMS Clinic at their university, which planned to use the Moos Menstrual Distress Questionnaire. He admitted that he had never tried it out on himself, so I dug one out and, with his wife's help he tried to complete it – or at least the bits which also apply to men. Maybe it was the effect of their recent jet flight, but the couple had the greatest difficulty in agreeing on even four questions, such as 'Have you been confused today?', 'Have you been forgetful today?'

Volunteers for trials are expected to complete no fewer than 47 such questions every night for six months, which means including holidays, occasional flu and migraine attacks and after a night out! Sampson's 1988 study enrolled 215 women, but only

69 women successfully completed the daily questionnaire. We are left wondering, were the 69 women really properly completing their nightly tasks, or did they cheat occasionally? Were they abnormally obsessive and introverted? To put it quite bluntly: were they normal, typical women? I don't think I'd be able to do all that recording properly for a full six months.

That brings us on to the next problem, which is the high number of women who initially enrol in the trials, but then drop out. It is always difficult to know how they should be counted. Did they stop because of the daily chore of completing the questionnaires, because of side effects, because they got worse or because they got better?

All trials on PMS have shown a high placebo response. That means that during the first month of having either the active drug or the placebo, all the patients in the study improve. Why? There are many suggested reasons, but no consensus of opinion. In 1982 three London gynaecologists, A. L. Magos, M. Brincot and J. W. W. Studd, studied the effect of implants in 68 women. They either gave a normal oestrogen implant or just anaesthetized the skin, cut the usual incision and sewed the skin back without inserting an oestrogen pellet. They reported that after the first month, 94 per cent of those who received the fake implant treatment improved. Unfortunately the effects of placebos don't last very long – if they did, we'd just use sugar or chalk pills instead of all these expensive drugs! Anyway, statisticians calculate that, because of this high placebo response, any successful PMS trial will need at least 120 women to complete a six-month study.

In Britain, clinical trials are carefully controlled and permission must be granted from the ethical committee of the hospital or the area health committee. The ethical committee must see a *protocol* showing precisely which patients are to be included and excluded, and the information the volunteers are to be given about the trials, together with a copy of the consent form which all women will be asked to sign before entering the trials.

Table 6 lists the special problems with PMS trials. Serious PMS patients must be excluded, which means those at risk or with a previous history of suicide, violence, fits, self-mutilation, alcoholic bouts, criminal acts or hospital admission. Volunteers must not be receiving any medication, including the Pill or vitamins, for the duration of the trials. Trials usually last six months: for the first two months the volunteer merely updates her monthly chart and the daily questionnaire each day. She will then be allotted to a treatment group, and will either receive an active drug or an inactive placebo for two months, and then she will change over and have two months of the other course of treatment. She will know before she agrees to participate that she will only receive treatment for two of the six months. So, for ethical reasons, double-blind crossover clinical trials must be limited to mild sufferers, whose symptoms are in fact so mild that they do not mind putting up with them for at least four of the next six months.

Table 6: Problems with PMS Trials

- Precise definition of PMS, with absence of symptoms in the postmenstruum
- High dropout rate
- High placebo response
- Long duration, at least six months of daily recording
- High number of volunteers required
- Numerous symptoms, both psychological and physical
- Limited to mild cases for ethical reasons
- No hormonal contraception
- No medication, prescribed or over the counter, for the duration of the trials

---

So far there has only been one well-controlled double-blind crossover trial of progesterone suppositories which met all the requirements and used an adequate dose of progesterone – this showed the benefit of progesterone over placebo. The British Multicentred General Practitioner Trial used 400 mg Cyclogest suppositories twice daily for the two treatment months. The authors are currently negotiating the next hurdle, which is to get the trial published in a reputable medical journal. This is not as easy as it sounds.

PMS IS NOW ACCEPTED IN LAW

On the other hand it is important to appreciate that PMS is accepted in English courts of law. Legal history was made in England in 1979 in a case of arson, *R. v. Owens*, and in 1980 in the cases of *R. v. Craddock* and *R. v. English* in regard to murder. Since then there have been many other cases and other crimes in which PMS was accepted as causing diminished responsibility or as a mitigating factor. It is usual for the defendant to plead guilty, and she is then given a probation order ensuring that she continues treatment for a stated length of time. If PMS is involved in a crime, then it is judged as being severe enough to require progesterone treatment. There has been at least one case to my knowledge in which the probation order stated that the defendant should give to the nurse who administered the progesterone injections a full written list of all food she had eaten during the previous day.

THE NHS TRIBUNAL ON OVERPRESCRIBING

The National Health Service in Britain was introduced in 1948. In those days, general practitioners had full freedom with the drugs they could prescribe, but to prevent unnecessary prescribing, each doctor received annually a statement of his or her prescribing costs and the number of prescriptions he or she had issued over a sample period of one month. Those whose prescription costs were considered too high were visited by a Ministry of Health official, who gently advised which cheaper drugs could be prescribed instead. If the doctor's prescription charges remained high for the next two years, he or she had to appear before the Family Practitioners Committee, who could decide whether the prescription costs were reasonable, and both the doctor or the Minister of Health could appeal against the decision of the Committee, in which case the problem would be left to be sorted out by a tribunal.

Progesterone Is a Reasonable and Necessary Treatment for PMS

In 1957 I was a general practitioner in Edmonton, Middle-sex, and had twice been visited by a man from the Ministry of Health because of my many prescriptions for progesterone injections for PMS sufferers. My heavy prescribing of progesterone continued, and I was called to appear before the doctors on the executive committee. I went armed with precise details of the 53 women to whom I had prescribed progesterone for PMS during the month in question. The details showed how money had, in fact, been saved by avoiding hospital admissions, sick pay, costs of home helps, ambulances and so on. This list of patients included many who had taken part in my study of PMS, published with Dr Raymond Greene in the *British Medical Journal* in 1953. The committee agreed that *progesterone was reasonable and necessary treatment for PMS*, but the Minister of Health appealed against the decision. In accordance with the NHS Act, the first ever Tribunal on Overprescribing was convened in 1958, with a barrister, a general practitioner from Birmingham and the Professor of Obstetrics from Liverpool University, and I was ably defended by the Medical Defence Union. The tribunal decided in my favour. Progesterone was *'reasonable and necessary' treatment for PMS*. They did add that mine was an overwhelmingly female practice; if all doctors prescribed a lot of progesterone for a long time, the price of progesterone injections would come down; but that if all doctors did prescribe progesterone at its present price to all their PMS patients, the drug bill would exceed the nation's defence budget!

Chapter 15

THE 'BEST BUYS'

Perhaps it is not surprising that a disease which has over 100 symptoms will also tend to have 100 different suggested treatments. Until there is a definitive diagnostic test to separate the 'haves' from the 'have nots' in PMS, there is unlikely to be only one 'best buy'. However, I hope that all women will realize that there is plenty of help available and that they are not alone. Hands are stretching out to help your misery: go out and find help during your 'good' days in the postmenstruum and don't be afraid to talk to your doctor about it. Nowadays he or she is unlikely to think it is 'all in your mind'.

We are all so different, not only in where we live and in our homes and dress, but also in age, race, weight and temperament. We all have our pet likes and dislikes when it comes to food, work, leisure and ways of socializing. All these factors have to be considered in choosing the 'best buy' for you personally.

DR DALTON'S STORY

My choice of best buys is the result of many years specializing in PMS and its many related illnesses. I have either tried, or heard at first-hand from patients who have experienced them, the many and various suggestions contained in this book. The only exception is colour therapy (Chapter 5), and personally I'm still not sure that one is not a leg-pull.

In 1948 I was a newly-qualified doctor doing my first locum job in a general practice. I was called out in the early hours one morning to a woman with severe asthma. Her husband met me at the door and apologized for calling me out at such an unearthly hour, but added, 'It happens every month; the only time she's well is when she's pregnant.'

These words rang a bell. I had recently been relieved of my own premenstrual migraine by progesterone, and the only time I had been completely free of it was during my three pregnancies. I saw the endocrinologist Dr Raymond Greene, who had helped me with my migraine, and together we discussed the possibility that such a thing as 'premenstrual asthma' might exist. In those days, doctors would have fallen about laughing at such an idea. (Some did just that, later on, including a London Professor of Medicine, author of the most popular textbook for students. In 1952, at the Royal Society of Medicine, he had the whole audience laughing at the ludicrous idea that women might have menstrual migraine, since men do not menstruate at all. However, few doctors if any would doubt its existence now.) Anyway, Dr Greene suggested I tried progesterone from ovulation to menstruation for my patient with premenstrual asthma next month.

During the following month I came across another woman with asthma, two with migraine and two with epilepsy; all claimed that their attacks only came before menstruation and all had been well during pregnancies. They also agreed to have progesterone injections. To everyone's delight, the progesterone worked and their unbelievable freedom from attacks brought happiness not only to the six women but also started Dr Greene and myself on a long journey of discovery. At that time it was not the psychological problems that interested us so much as the monthly attacks of bodily symptoms. My deep interest in PMS continued during my 20-odd years in general practice, followed by over 25 years in a consultant practice dealing only with PMS and related diseases. There have been trials and tribulations on the way, but today, with all the plethora of possible treatments, one can promise hope and help to all.

THE BEST BUYS

The first essential is to decide whether the problem is in fact caused by PMS, and the only way to do this is to chart the daily symptoms and the dates of menstruation (Chapter 1).

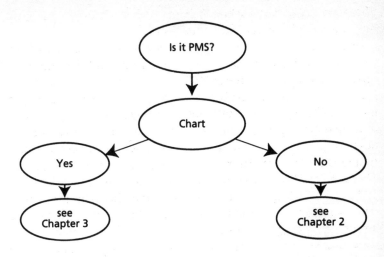

Figure 47: Is it PMS?

If the chart suggests that it is not PMS, all is not lost; Chapter 2 may give you some clues and help you decide where to go from here.

For all PMS sufferers, whether their symptoms are mild, moderate or drastically severe, my first recommendation would be to learn and practise the coping skills (Chapter 5). Look at your menstrual chart, enjoy your postmenstruum and arrange

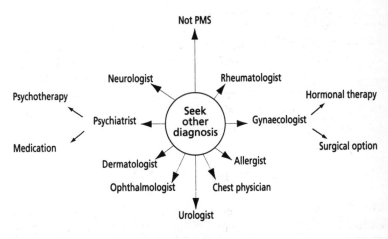

Figure 48: It's Not PMS

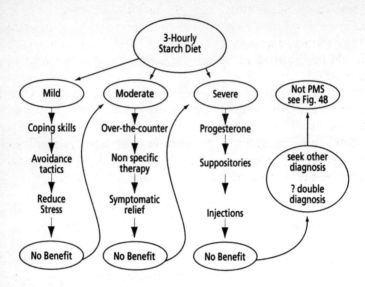

Figure 49: It is PMS

appointments at the right time so that you can have the deserved peace and quietness at the awkward times. This is something that you, your partner and family can do together, so share your misery. There are plenty who want to help, if they only know how. Tell them and help them to understand your plight and your desire to be well.

The next best buy, which again is needed regardless of how mild or severe your affliction, is to follow religiously the three-hourly starch diet (Chapter 6) throughout the entire month. This entails no financial outlay, but does demand self-discipline and determination. The effort brings worthwhile rewards.

Again, get others to understand and help your 'clock-watching'; then they won't mistake your constant nibbling for greed. Get the children to remind you when time's up. Children would much prefer a nibbling diet to the strict no-food-between-meals rule. Even if progesterone therapy is needed, it is still essential to maintain the three-hourly starch diet.

Finally, for the severe sufferers who have not benefited sufficiently from the coping skills and the three-hourly starch diet, the best buy is progesterone (Chapter 11) – making sure that the rules of progesterone therapy are followed to the letter.

While suppositories will benefit the majority of severe sufferers, there are always a few who will need intramuscular injections. This treatment has stood the test of time and today, as in 1958, it should be regarded as 'reasonable and necessary treatment for PMS' (Chapter 14).

PMS is a chronic, or long-term, disease, and the tendency for it to develop will be present until the menopause. Be warned that its severity will increase at times of stress, when weight reducing and when doing night work. Caution is advised against drastic irreversible treatments such as hysterectomy and/or oophorectomy, before reaching menopausal age (Chapter 11).

DAVID HOLTON'S BEST BUY

I would also recommend all of the above (Dr Dalton has grabbed all the best ones), leaving me with but one recommendation (but it's a good one!):
Send a stamped, addressed envelope to:

PMS Help
PO Box 160
St Albans
Herts AL1 4UQ

This is an organization which I helped to set up some years ago, and I am still on the committee. They will offer you membership, which includes free postal advice and a regular newsletter with readers' letters, hints and tips plus all the latest on research into PMS. They have a good range of booklets at very reasonable prices, as well as a lot of books (such as this one!) and you can even buy their own, professionally produced and award-winning video, *PMS Steps to Freedom*, for under £10.

PMS Help booklets
- What is PMS?
- Can Diet help your PMS?
- Too Young for PMS?
- Do Men suffer from PMS?

What is more, by joining PMS Help you will help them in their work of educating the medical profession, the media and the general public about PMS and related hormonal diseases, as well as furthering medical research into the subject. The charity recognizes that as well as helping individual sufferers with their troubles, and providing support for them, much wider action is needed to get the problem properly under control.

Dr Dalton is one of the many distinguished patrons of PMS Help, and contributes regularly to the newsletter.

It saddens me greatly to have to say this, but at the time of writing neither Dr Dalton nor I know of any other good national organization for PMS. Be especially suspicious of those which aren't registered charities; they tend to want lots of money for dubious advice or treatments. In fact, before you accept anything regarding PMS, here or abroad, find out how much money is involved.

For those at their wits' end, who feel that no one has ever suffered as badly as them before, may I suggest they read the book *Nicola* by Nicola Owen (Corgi Books, 1993). It is the true story of Nicola Owen, who was a beautiful, talented dancer at 14 years of age but who, over the next four years, developed extreme mood swings with suicide attempts, self-mutilation and bizarre actions, including swallowing weedkiller, and arson. She ended up in Holloway Prison charged with arson and endangering life, with the possibility of going to Broadmoor (an institution for insane criminals). Then PMS was diagnosed and progesterone treatment started. She made legal history in 1979 when PMS was first recognized in an English Court and she was released on probation. Today she is once again a self-confident, beautiful, composed, healthy married woman, who has literally lived happily ever after.

GLOSSARY

Abdomen the body's cavity between the diaphragm and the pelvis, containing the stomach, intestines, liver, pancreas, kidneys, ureter and bladder

Abortion death of fetus

Acne spots on the skin due to blocking of the sebaceous glands

Adrenal glands two glands situated above the kidneys and responsible for producing numerous hormones

Adrenalin one of the hormones produced by the adrenal glands

Afterbirth see **Placenta**

Allergy unusual reaction produced in certain individuals to specific items, e.g. foods, pollens

Amenorrhoea absence of menstruation

Anaemia insufficient iron in the blood

Analgesic drug taken to relieve pain

Anorexia loss of appetite

Anorexia nervosa a disease characterized by loss of appetite, weight loss and, in women, cessation of menstruation

Anovular without ovulation

Antenatal during pregnancy and before childbirth

Antidepressant drug to remove depression

Antihistamine drug which counteracts the effects of histamine, which is released in allergic reactions

Anus exit from alimentary canal, or back passage

Aromatherapy treatment with fragrant oils

Atypical not typical

Bromocriptine a drug which reduces prolactin levels

Candida a yeast normally present in the alimentary canal

Cervical smear test for the diagnosis of cancer of the womb
Cervix entrance to the womb
Chromosomes tiny threadlike structures within the cell nucleus, containing genes
Conception becoming pregnant by fertilization of the ovum
Contraception prevention of pregnancy
Corticosteroids hormones produced by the adrenal cortex
Cystitis inflammation of the urinary bladder
Diuretics drugs which increase the output of urine
Dysmenorrhoea pain with menstruation
Dyspareunia pain on intercourse
ECT electroconvulsive therapy, in which an electric shock is administered to the brain
Embryo developing ovum up to the end of the eighth week after conception
Endocrine glands organs releasing hormones into the blood to act on some other part of the body
Endocrinologist a person studying the hormones of the body
Endogenous arising from within
Endometrium inner lining of the womb
Exogenous arising from without
Fallopian tubes two tubes from the ovaries to the womb along which the egg cells pass
Fetus developing baby in the womb
Follicle stimulating hormone (FSH) hormone produced by the pituitary to act on the ovary to ripen the follicles and stimulate the ovary to produce oestrogen
Follicular phase days after menstruation and before ovulation, when the follicle stimulating hormone is active
Galactorrhoea milk from the breasts when not breastfeeding
Genes factors controlling heredity carried by chromosomes
Geriatric medicine care of the elderly
Glaucoma disease of the eye characterized by increased pressure in the eye
Glucose a form of sugar found in the blood
Gonadotrophin hormone from the pituitary acting on the gonads (either the testes or ovaries)
Gonadotrophin releasing hormone (GnRH) hormone from hypothalamus to the pituitary which stimulates the gonads (ovaries in women)

Gonads sexual organs, either testes or ovaries

Gynaecology the study of diseases of women

Haemorrhage loss of blood, bleeding

Homoeopathy treatment by drugs which produce in the patient the symptoms of the disease to be cured, but which are given in very minute doses

Hormone chemical messenger produced by glands and having an action on cells in another part of the body

Hyperglycaemia raised blood sugar level

Hyperthyroidism excessive thyroid activity

Hypnosis an artificially produced state resembling sleep

Hypnotic drug to induce sleep

Hypoglycaemia lowered blood sugar level

Hypothalamus part of the base of the brain containing the control centres

Hypothyroidism underactive thyroid function

Hysterectomy removal of the womb

Implant pellet of a drug inserted into the tissues

Infanticide killing of an infant by its mother

Intermenstrual the days between menstruation and the premenstruum, usually days 5 to 24 of the cycle

Intra-uterine device (IUD) small contraceptive device inserted into the womb

Iron an essential mineral required by the red cells of the blood. Insufficient iron causes anaemia

Labour birth of baby

Lactation breastfeeding

Laparoscopy examination of the abdomen by periscope

Laparotomy direct visual examination of the abdomen through a surgical incision

Lethargy excessive tiredness

Libido sex drive

Lithium a metal normally present in the body only in minute traces

Luteinizing hormone (LH) hormone produced by the pituitary, which stimulates ovulation and the production of progesterone

Luteinizing phase that part of the menstrual cycle under the influence of the luteinizing hormone, namely from ovulation to menstruation

Magnesium   a mineral required by the body in only minute amounts

Mania   mental illness marked by unusual elation or excessive activity

Maternity   related to pregnancy

Menarche   first menstruation

Menopause   last menstruation

Menorrhagia   heavy menstrual bleeding

Menstrual controlling centre   situated in the hypothalamus and responsible for the cyclical timing of menstruation

Menstrual loss   bleeding at menstruation

Menstruation   monthly bleeding from the vagina in women of reproductive age, caused by disintegration of the lining of the womb

Metabolism   building up and breaking down of the chemicals of the body

Migraine   severe form of headache

Mittelschmerz   abdominal pain at the time of ovulation

Nucleus   central vital part of every living cell, where metabolism occurs

Obstetrician   doctor specializing in the care of women during pregnancy and labour

Oestrogen   hormone released by the ovary

Oophorectomy   removal of an ovary

Ovary   reproductive organ containing egg cells

Ovulation   release of egg cell from ovum

Ovum   egg cell

Paramenstruum   the days immediately before menstruation and days of menstruation

Parturition   birth of baby

Pituitary   gland situated immediately below the brain, producing numerous hormones

Placebo   inert or inactive substance which has no curative effect

Placenta   organ which develops during pregnancy within the womb and is responsible for feeding the fetus and for the production of hormones

Postmenstruum   the days immediately after menstruation

Postnatal   after childbirth

Potassium   mineral present in the blood and cells of the body

Pre-eclampsia illness in late pregnancy characterized by high blood pressure, water retention and protein in the urine

Premenstruum days before menstruation

Preovulatory days before ovulation

Progesterone hormone produced by the ovary for the preparation of the lining of the womb, for the maintenance of pregnancy and the starting-point for the production of numerous corticosteroids

Progestin American name for progestogen

Progestogen man-made steroid capable of causing bleeding from the lining of the womb, and having different actions to that of natural progesterone

Prolactin hormone produced by the pituitary; its most important function is in breastfeeding

Prophylactic preventative

Psychosis mental illness

Puerperium the days after childbirth

Pyrexia fever

Pyridoxine Vitamin B_6

Sedative drug to bring calmness

Sodium essential mineral present in the blood and cells

Spasmodic dysmenorrhoea spasms of pain with menstruation

Sterile incapable of becoming pregnant

Sterilization operation to permanently prevent pregnancy

Stress the reaction to the demands made upon a person

Symptoms complaints of ill health

Synchrony occurring at the same time

Syndrome collection of symptoms which commonly occur together

Testes two male reproductive organs which produce sperm and testosterone

Testosterone male hormone produced by the testes

Therapy treatment

Thyroid gland in the neck producing hormones responsible for the speed of metabolism in the body

Tranquillizer drug to bring tranquillity

Trauma injury to body or mind

Uterus womb

Vagina passage from the womb to the outside of the body

Vaginitis inflammation of the vagina

Vasectomy surgical operation on a man to make him permanently sterile

Vitamins substances contained in food essential for life, growth and reproduction

Yeast vegetable microorganism normally present and harmless when in the alimentary canal, but can cause thrush if in the vagina or mouth

Zinc a mineral required by the body, but only in a very minute quantity

FURTHER READING

Once A Month, K Dalton (Fontana, 1991)

Premenstrual Syndrome Illustrated, K Dalton (Peter Andrew of Droitwich, 1990)

Premenstrual Syndrome Goes to Court, K Dalton (Peter Andrew of Droitwich, 1990)

Premenstrual Syndrome – How to beat It, Ian Simpson and Wendy Holton (Peter Andrew of Droitwich, 1992)

Premenstrual Syndrome Special Diet Cookbook, Jill Davies (Thorsons, 1991)

Depression After Childbirth, K Dalton, (Oxford University Press, 1989)

Nicola – The case that made legal history, N Owen (Bantam Press, 1992)

USEFUL ADDRESSES

PMS Help,
PO Box 160,
St Albans,
Herts AL1 4UQ

Amarant Trust,
16-24 Lonsdale Road
London NW6 6RD

Association of Postnatal Illness
25 Jerdan Place,
Fulham,
London SW6 1BE

British Migraine Association,
178a High Road,
Byfleet,
West Byfleet,
Surrey KT14 7ED

Endometriosis Society,
65 Holmedene Avenue
Herne Hill,
London SE24

Hysterectomy Support Network,
3 Lynn Close,
Green Street Green,
Orpington
Kent BR6 6BG

Meet-A-Mum-Association,
14 Illis Road,
Croydon
Surrey CR0 2XX

Migraine Trust,
45 Great Ormond Street,
London WC1N 3HZ

Miscarriage Association,
c/o Clayton Hospital,
Northgate,
Wakefield,
Yorks WF1 3JS

National Childbirth Trust,
Alexandra House
Oldham Terrace,
London W3 6NH

National Osteoporosis Society,
PO Box 10
Radstock,
Bath BA3 3YB

Relaxation for Living,
168-70 Oatlands Drive,
Weybridge,
Surrey KT13 9ET

SADA [Seasonal Affective Disorder Association]
51 Bracewell Road
London W10 6AF

SANDS [Stillbirth and Neonatal Deaths Society]
28 Portland Place,
London W1N 4DF

Index

Abdominal pain 34
Acne 82, 140
Acupuncture 86
Adolescents 13
Adopted daughters 15
Adrenal gland 45, 53
Adrenalin 69, 70, 71, 114
Agitation 78
Aggression 31, 32, 35, 71
AIDS 158
Alcohol 14, 16, 66, 67, 78 93, 128, 171
Aldactone 114
Allergy 79, 80, 104
Allergists 36
Alzheimer's disease 98
Anaemia 170
Anafranil 109
Analgesic 105, 162
Angina 89
Animals 53, 56
Anne of Cleves xviii
Anovular cycles 21
Anticonvulsant 114, 115
Antidepressant 7, 54, 106, 108, 109, 110, 162
Anxiety 33, 35, 55, 69, 71, 78, 83

Appetite 108
Arachis oil 128
Arithmetic 154
Aromatherapy 86
Arson 173, 180
Art therapy 88
Aspirin 104, 105, 106
Assertiveness 83
Asthma 29, 33, 36, 53, 81, 114, 151, 175, 176
Athletes 132
Ativan 112
Attack form 30
Aventyl 109
Avoidance tactics 60

Baby blues 24
Backache 36, 87, 115, 151
Bach flower remedy 88
Ballet dancers 132
Bamford 100
Barbiturates 112
Behavioural therapy 85
Benzodiazepines 112, 113
Berth-Jones 100
Betablockers 112, 113
Binges 15, 36, 73, 74, 82
Bio-energetics 88

191

Bladder 53
Bladderwort 101
Blaustein J D 51, 123
Bloatedness, 14, 21, 35, 69, 79, 82, 113, 163
Blood pressure 104, 150, 151, 153, 158, 167
Blood sugar level 50, 53, 69, 70, 72, 74, 79, 122, 123, 167
Bones 53, 87, 101
    pains 33
    mineral density 133
Breasts 100
    feeding 158
    swelling 113
    tenderness 21, 33, 36, 82
Brufen 105
Bulimia 132
Burinex 114

Caffeine 77, 78, 105, 106
Calcium 99
Camomile tea 113
Cancer 81, 144
Candida 78, 128
Candidiasis 78
Canestan 128
Carbohydrates 69, 72, 73
Cardiac physician 36
Catherine the Great xvi
Celest 136
Cervix 142
Cheese 72
Chest physician 36
Childbirth 5
Children 154, 155, 156
Chocolates 72, 73, 79, 108
Chorionic gonadotrophin 45
Chromium 98

Citrus fruit 79
Clauberg test 134
Clinical trials 171
    protocols 171
Cocaine 100
Codeine 105, 106
Coffee 73, 77, 78
Cognitive therapy 85
Conception 147
Confusion 71
Condom 160
Cola 78
Colour therapy 67, 175
Committee of Safety of Medicines 87, 90, 91, 100, 125
Conjunctivitis 36
Contraception 139, 158
Contraceptive pill 65, 158, 162, 163
Convulsions 152
Cortisone 53, 119
Counselling 84
Crime 173
Criminal acts 171
Criminals 38
Cyclogest 125, 172
Cyprus 125
Cystitis 36, 82, 115
Cytoplasm 50

D & C 116, 141, 142
Dairy products 79
Danazol 139, 140, 146, 165
Dandelion 101
Davies J 97
Day/Night Rhythm 44, 62
Defective luteal phase 148
Dental surgeon 36

Depression 14, 25, 31, 35, 37, 55, 69, 71, 81, 82, 107, 108, 109
  manic 111
  postnatal 156, 157, 158
Dermatologists 36, 100, 115
Diabetes 5, 38, 73, 93, 169, 170
Diagnosis 6, 12
Diarrhoea 99, 127, 160
Diet 59, 69
Diflucan 78, 128
Digitalis 100
Distalgesic 106
Dopamine 54
Dothiapin 109
Double blind cross over trials 168
Dowager's hump 99, 132
Duphaston 136, 137, 170
Dydrogesterone 136, 137, 169, 170
Dysmenorrhoea 18, 21, 81, 140
  congestive 21, 22, 23
  secondary 21
  spasmodic 21, 22, 23, 83, 139, 142

Eczema 100
Eggs 72
Embryo 43, 148
Endocrinologists 3, 176
Endometrial resection 144
Endometriosis 18, 23, 140, 144
English 154
Equigesic 105
Epilepsy 114, 151, 152
Ethidronate 133

Ethisterone 138
Ethyloleate 128
EUA 141, 142
Examinations 155
Exercise 63, 64
Eye 53, 81, 104, 113

Fainting 21, 152
Fallopian tubes 53, 143
Faverin 112
Feel-Well Factor 82
Fibroids 144
Fish 72
Fits 171
Flour 71
Flurazepam 112
Fluconazole 78
Follicle stimulating hormone 27, 45, 47
Folic acid 102
Forgetfulness 25
Frumil 114

Gamma linoleic acid 99
Gastroenterologist 115
Garlic tablets 40, 103
Genetic factors 15
General Practitioners 134, 158, 163, 166, 167
Ginseng 102
Gonadotrophin Releasing Hormones 44, 45, 134, 146
  Agonists 140
  Antagonists 140
Ground ivy 101
Gynaecology 6
Gynaecologists 7, 116, 134, 136, 142, 144, 163, 171

Haemophilia 5
Hay fever 36
Heart 104
Headache 14, 21, 36, 82, 101, 104, 147, 151, 152, 153
Heart failure 81
Henry VIII xviii
Hexonoate 136
Hippocrates xvii
HIV 158
Holton W M 75
Homeopathy 88
Hong Kong 125
Hormone 45, 50
    receptors 49
    test 119
HRT 28, 137, 138, 144, 162, 163
Hot flushes 25
Hydrocortisone 119
Hydroxyprogesterone 136
Hyperemesis 149, 158
Hyperinsulinaemia 47
Hypertension 99
Hypnotics 113
Hypoglycaemia 74
Hypon 105
Hypothalamus 17, 62, 140
Hypothyroidism 5
Hysterectomy 138, 140, 141, 144, 145, 146, 165, 170, 179

Ibuprofen 105
Immunoglobulin 79
Imipramine 109
Inderal 113
Indocid 105
Indomethacin 105
Inhalers 114

Insomnia 55, 78, 108, 110
Insulin 118, 169, 170
Intelligence 53, 155
In Vitro Fertilization (IVF) 42, 121, 148, 155
Iron 98, 99
Irrationality 35
Irritability 21, 31, 32, 35, 63, 69, 71, 81, 108

Kidneys 45, 48, 62, 104, 105, 106, 113
Kidney failure 81
Kleinjen J L 94
Korea 125

Lactation 46
Lamentations xvi
Laparoscopy 6, 116, 143, 167
Laparectomy 143
Lasix 114
Law 172
Levonorgestrel 136
Lethargy 35
Liver 48
Lorazepam 112
Luteal phase 52
Lutineizing hormone 45, 140
Lustral 112

Magnesium 97, 98
Magos A L 171
Maize 71
Moniliasis 128
Malaria 88
Manic depression 111
Marce 25
Marriage guidance counsellor 84
Marilyn Monroe xviii

Marker, Russell 119
Masculinization 140
MAST test 79
Maternal behaviour 55
Meadowsweet 101
Meat 72
Medicine Control Agency 101
Medical Defence Union 174
Medroxyprogesterone acetate 136
Mefenamic Acid 105, 106
Menopause 7, 16, 18, 25, 27, 28, 87, 121, 130, 132, 137, 146, 163, 179
Menorrhagia 144
Menstrual
  controlling centre 44, 62, 144, 146
  chart 8, 10, 11, 12, 19, 20, 23, 27, 122, 145, 163, 176, 177
  distress 18, 19, 77, 104
  magnification 19, 77, 104
Menstruation 9, 43, 44, 46, 47, 116, 131, 145, 156, 157, 158, 159, 176
Mice 55
Midamore 114
Midwife 156
Migraine 29, 36, 80, 87, 101, 151, 170, 176
  classical 29
Miscarriage 121, 148, 149, 150
Mittleschmerz 138
Moduretic 114
Mogadon 113
Monoamine Oxidase Inhibitors (MAOIs) 54, 66, 110

Mood control 44
Mood swings 21, 35
MOOS Menstrual Distress Questionnaire 170
Morning sickness 121, 149
Motherwort 101
Motrin 105
Multiple sclerosis 98
Multivitamin 96
Murder 173

Nausea 14, 34, 36, 152
Neogest 136
Niacin 102
Nicola 180
Nicotine 66
Night sweats 25
  work 16, 62
Nitrazepam 112, 113
Nock B 50
Nonsteroidal anti-inflammatory drugs (NSAID) 105, 162
Norethiderol 136
Norethisterone 136, 138
Norgeston 136
Nucleus 50, 69
Nurofen 105
Numbness 94
Nymphomania 15, 108

Oats 71
Obstetricians 153, 156
Oestradiol 132
Oestrogens, 27, 45, 53, 87, 119, 130, 132, 133, 134, 139, 145, 162
  implants 139, 171
  patches 139
  tablets 139

Oestrone 132

Oil of Evening Primrose 99, 100

Oophorectomy 141, 146, 179

Ophthalmologist 36, 115

Opium 100

Oral progesterone 124

Osteopathy 87

Osteoporosis 99, 132, 133, 137, 138, 140, 163

Otologist 36, 115

Ovaries 118, 143, 144

Ovary 27, 45, 53, 140

Over the Counter medicines 90, 161, 164, 165, 172

Ovid xvi

Ovulation 176

Ovum 43

Pancreas 45

Panic 71, 80, 82

Paranoia 35

Paracodol 106

Paracetamol 104, 105, 106, 167

Paroxitine 112

Parnate 110

Parsley 101

Parstelin 110

Passiflora 101

Peripheral neuritis 93

Pethidine 105

Phobias 85

Phosphorus 98

Physical education 154

Physicians 3, 115

Pill - contraceptive 5, 13, 42, 65, 117, 125, 135, 137, 165

Pituitary 140

glands 45

Placebo 82, 168, 169, 171, 172

Placenta 43, 45, 123, 148, 149

PMS Help 40, 179

Polyps 142

Postmenstruum 175

Ponstan 105, 106

Postnatal depression 18, 24, 47, 54, 55, 121, 125, 156, 157, 158

Potassium 98, 114

Potato 71

Pregnancy 47, 147, 150, 152, 176

Pregnanediol 47

Premenstruum 61, 63, 66, 83, 84, 86

Primulut N 136

Probation 173

Propranalol 113

Progesterone 44, 45, 47, 50, 52, 53, 54, 55, 56, 66, 69, 72, 116, 120, 121, 123, 124, 133, 135, 138, 145, 146, 149, 150, 151, 153, 155, 156, 158, 162, 163, 173

blood levels 52, 54, 120, 121, 126, 136, 147, 158

contraception 159, 160

implants 122, 130

injections 116, 122, 125, 126, 128, 129, 130, 131, 135, 157, 174, 179

micronised 124

oral 124

pessaries 122, 125

receptors 6, 50, 51, 52, 54, 69, 117, 118, 136, 144

suppositories 116, 122, 124, 125, 126, 128, 131, 157
suspension 127
treatment 116, 131, 173, 174, 178, 179, 180
Progestogens 14, 119, 120, 121, 122, 134, 135, 137, 138, 139, 140, 153, 158, 162, 163, 164, 166
Progestins 134
Prolactin 47
Prostaglandin 106
Prostaglandin Inhibitors 105
Prothiaden 109
Provera 136
Prozac 112
Psychiatrists 3, 107
Psychotherapy 84
Puberty 5
Puerperal fever xiv
Pyridoxine 93, 162
overdose neuropathy 33, 93

Queen Elizabeth I xvi
Queen Victoria xvi
RAST blood test 79
Rats 55
Rebirthing 88
Reflexology 87
Relate Counsellor 84
Relaxation 63, 83
Rheumatologist 36, 115
Rhinitis 33, 53
Rickets 91
Rice 71
Rivofavin 102
Royal Jelly 102
Rye 71

Salad 72

Salt 79
Saluric 114
Sampson G 169
Sandwich 72
Schaumberg H 93
Scurvy 91
Seasonal Affective Disorder 29
Self help groups 64, 65
Self-hypnosis 85
Self-mutilation 35, 171, 180
Semelweiss xiii
Sex Hormone Binding Globulin 47, 48, 49
Sertraline 112
Shaitsu 88
Silva 88
Sinequin 112
Singapore 125
Sinusitis 53, 115
Skin 53, 81
Skullcap 101
Sleep 62, 101, 108
Slimming xviii
Smoking 16, 66, 78
Sodium 98, 114
Sore throat 34, 36, 53
South Africa 125
Spasmodic dysmenorrhoea - see dysmenorrhoea
Spironolactone 114
Starch 72, 74
Starflower oil 100
Stelazine 112
Sterilisation 13, 14, 132, 141, 143, 158, 165
Stress 101
Stress Medicine 75
Studd J 171
Suicide 171, 180
Sugar 72, 73, 74, 101

Solpadol 106
Surmontal 109
Symptoms 9

Tea 73, 77, 78
Teacher 61
Temazepam 112, 113
Temperature 53
Tenormin 113
Tension 35, 69, 77, 81, 108, 112
  Headache 29
Testosterone 53, 119, 130, 135, 146, 155
Thalidomide 41
Three Hourly Starch Diet 71, 75, 76, 77, 104, 114, 121, 123, 145, 165, 178
Thrush 122, 128
Thyroid 38, 48
Thyroxine 5
Tylex 106
Tiredness 21, 31, 32, 39, 63, 81, 109
Tofranil 109
Toxaemia of pregnancy 150, 152
Tranquillisers 7, 101, 110, 162
Tribunal on overprescribing 174
Triphasic 109
Tryptizol 109

Ultrasonic pelvic scan 6, 142, 148
Urethritis 115
Urologists 36, 115

Vasectomy 158
Vegetables 72
Venus xviii
Verbal reasoning 154, 155
Video 179
Violence 171
Vitamins 40, 48, 90, 91, 92, 93, 97, 103, 165
Vitamin B$_6$ 91, 93, 95, 98, 103, 162
  overdose 94
Vomiting 21, 36, 149, 150, 152

Wang M L 55
Water retention 113
Weight controlling centre 44
  gain 14, 38, 69, 70, 108, 140, 150, 153
  loss 108
  swings 15
Wheat 79

Yeast 78

Zinc 97